GUT CHECK
COOKBOOK

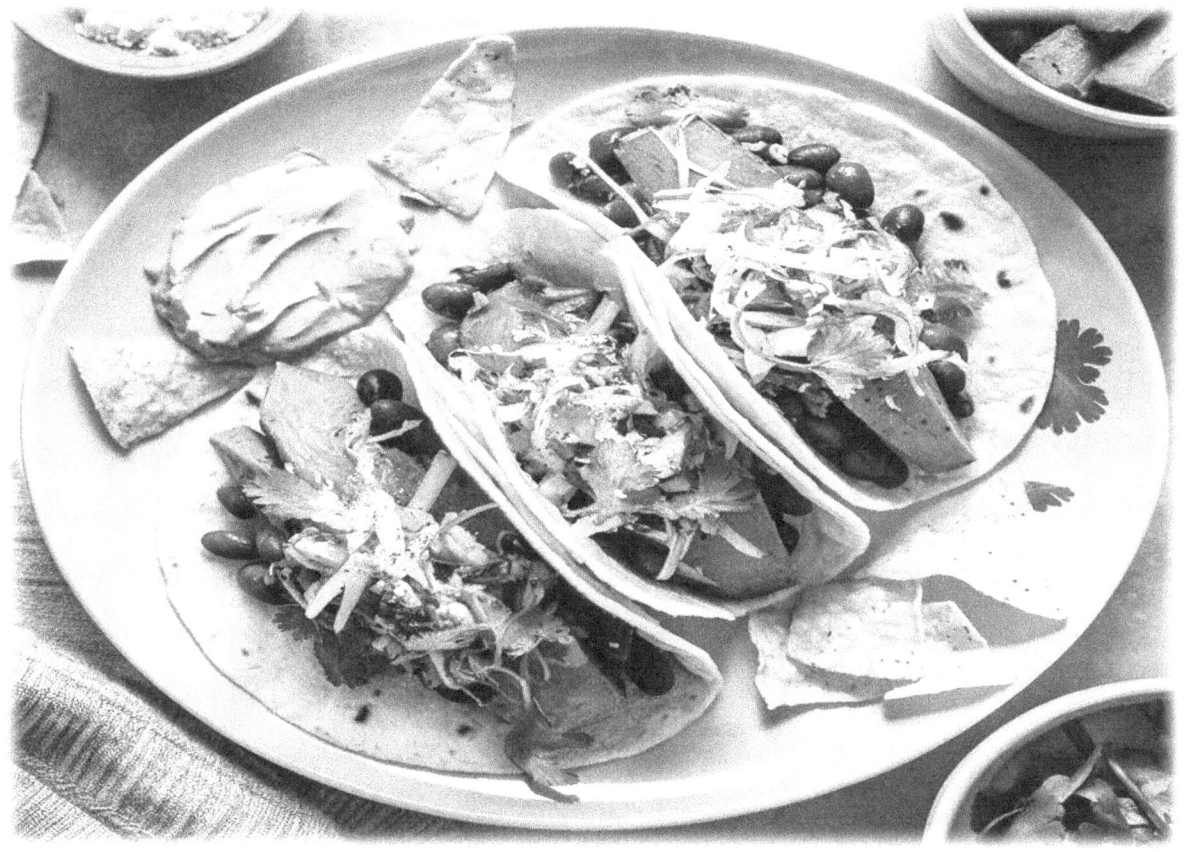

Relieve Gout Pain with Flavor: Essential Low-Purine Recipes and a 28-Day Meal Plan for Lasting Relief and Better Health"

Monalisa Blake

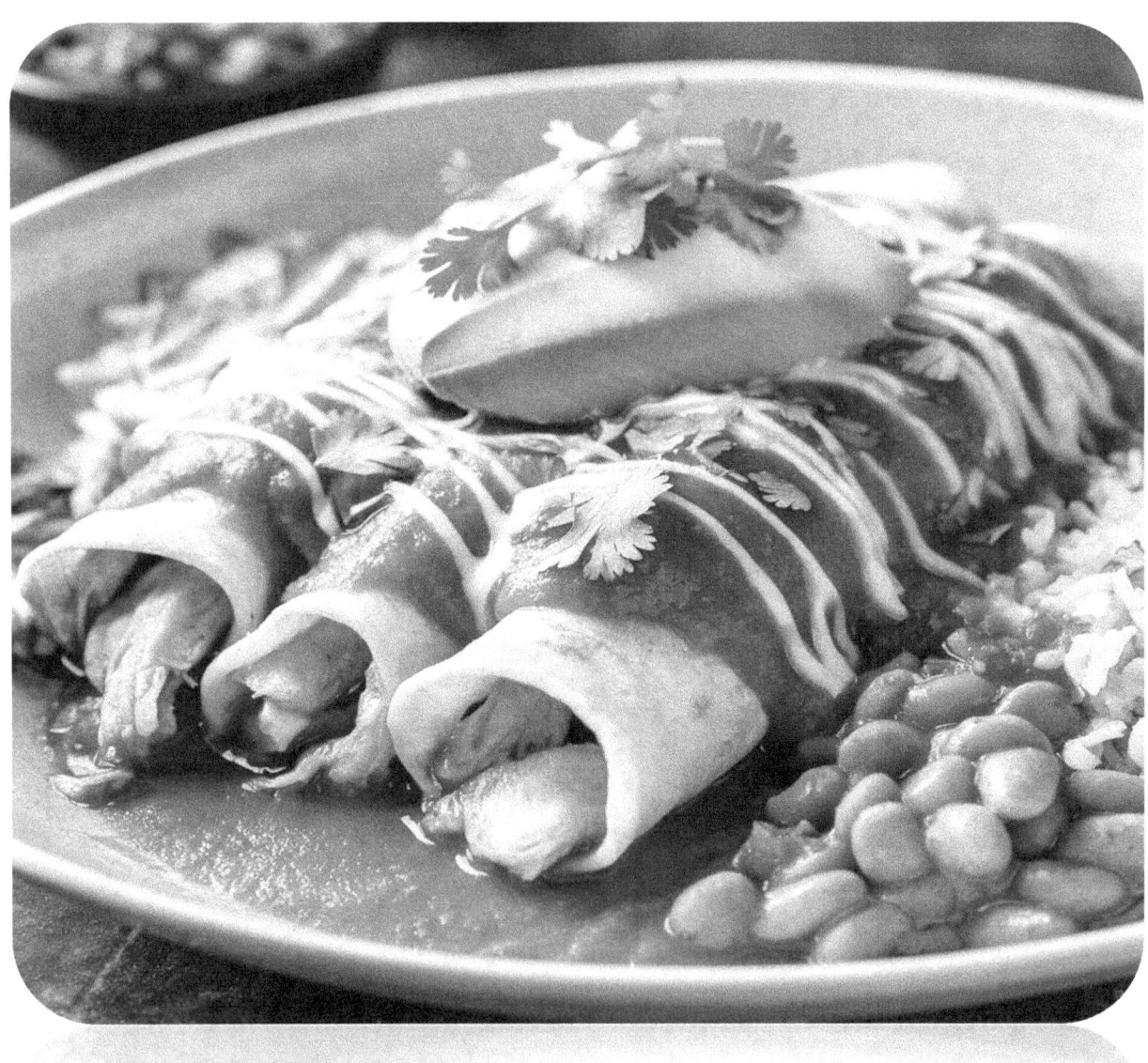

TABLE OF CONTENT

Introduction

Imagine a bustling farmer's market in the heart of Provence, France. The air is filled with the aroma of fresh herbs, the chatter of vendors, and the vibrant colors of fruits and vegetables. This picturesque scene is not just a feast for the senses but a testament to the profound connection between food, culture, and health. It's here that our journey into the world of gut health begins.

Just as the French have long cherished their local, seasonal produce, the principles of gut health are rooted in understanding the profound impact of what we consume on our overall well-being. The "GUT CHECK COOKBOOK" aims to bring this ancient wisdom into your kitchen, blending it with modern science to help you achieve a healthier, happier life.

The Importance of a Healthy Gut

Your gut, often referred to as your second brain, plays a crucial role in your overall health. From digestion and nutrient absorption to immune function and even mental health, the gut influences many aspects of our well-being. Recent studies have shown that a balanced gut microbiome can help reduce inflammation, improve mood, and even aid in weight management.

Yet, in today's fast-paced world, many of us struggle with gut health issues like bloating, indigestion, and food intolerances. This cookbook is designed to address these challenges by providing you with delicious, gut-friendly recipes and practical tips for maintaining a healthy digestive system.

Overview of Gut Health in the USA, Europe, and Globally

The quest for optimal gut health transcends borders. In the USA, the rise of processed foods and a sedentary lifestyle has led to a surge in digestive issues. Across Europe, traditional diets rich in fermented foods and fresh produce have long supported gut health, but modern influences are beginning to take their toll. Globally, the integration of diverse culinary traditions offers a wealth of knowledge and variety that can enhance our understanding and approach to gut health.

Importance and Overview

The Crucial Role of a Healthy Gut

Your gut, often referred to as your second brain, is more than just a part of your digestive system. It plays a pivotal role in maintaining your overall health. From breaking down the food you eat to absorbing essential nutrients and protecting your body from harmful pathogens, the gut is a powerhouse of activity. Recent scientific research has uncovered that a balanced gut microbiome— the trillions of bacteria and other microorganisms living in your digestive tract— is integral to your physical and mental well-being.

A healthy gut can reduce inflammation, enhance immune function, improve mental clarity, and even aid in weight management. Conversely, an imbalance in gut bacteria can lead to a host of problems, including digestive disorders, allergies, mental health issues, and chronic diseases. Understanding and nurturing your gut health is, therefore, a fundamental aspect of achieving overall wellness.

Global Perspectives on Gut Health

Gut health is a universal concern, but dietary habits and lifestyles vary widely across different regions, influencing how we approach it.

In the USA, the prevalence of processed foods and a sedentary lifestyle has led to a spike in digestive issues and related health problems. The Standard American Diet (SAD) is often criticized for its high sugar, fat, and low fiber content, which can disrupt the delicate balance of the gut microbiome. This cookbook aims to counteract these trends by introducing recipes rich in fiber, probiotics, and essential nutrients to help restore gut health.

Europe, with its diverse culinary traditions, offers a wealth of knowledge in gut-friendly eating. The Mediterranean diet, for example, is celebrated for its emphasis on whole grains, fresh vegetables, fruits, nuts, seeds, and olive oil— all of which support a healthy gut. Fermented foods like yogurt, sauerkraut, and kefir are staples in many European diets, providing natural probiotics that foster a balanced microbiome.

Globally, traditional diets from various cultures offer invaluable insights into maintaining gut health. From the miso soups and pickled vegetables of Japan to the rich, fermented dairy products of Central Asia, these time-honored practices underscore the importance of whole, natural foods in supporting digestive health. By incorporating these diverse culinary traditions, this cookbook provides a comprehensive approach to gut health that can be adapted to suit any palate.

How to Use This Cookbook

Welcome to the "GUT CHECK COOKBOOK," your comprehensive guide to achieving optimal gut health through delicious and nutritious meals. This cookbook is designed to be user-friendly, informative, and inspiring, providing you with the tools you need to transform your health from the inside out. Here's how to make the most of this resource:

Understanding the Structure

This cookbook is divided into several key sections, each focusing on different aspects of gut health and nutrition. Here's a quick overview:

1. **Introduction and Education:**

    o **Importance and Overview:** Learn about the critical role of gut health and its impact on your overall well-being.

    o **Understanding Your Gut and The Gut Microbiome:** Gain foundational knowledge about the gut's anatomy, functions, and the importance of a balanced microbiome.

2. **Gut-Friendly Recipes:**

    o **Breakfasts for a Better Gut:** Start your day with energizing and nourishing breakfast options.

    o **Lunches to Love Your Gut:** Enjoy balanced and fiber-rich lunches that support digestion.

    o **Dinner Delights for Digestion:** Discover hearty and satisfying dinners that are easy on your gut.

    o **Snack Smarter:** Find gut-boosting snacks for those in-between moments.

    o **Desserts That Do Good:** Indulge in sweet treats that are also beneficial for your digestive health.

3. **Special Diets for Gut Health:**

    o Explore tailored recipes for gluten-free, dairy-free, low-FODMAP, and plant-based diets, ensuring you can enjoy gut-friendly meals regardless of dietary restrictions.

4. **Meal Planning and Preparation:**

    o **Sample Weekly Plans:** Get inspired with sample meal plans to help you organize your week.

- o **Hydration and Gut-Friendly Beverages:** Learn about the importance of hydration and discover recipes for gut-healthy drinks.

5. **Lifestyle and Gut Health:**

   - o Understand the role of exercise, stress management, and sleep in maintaining a healthy gut.

6. **Regional and Global Specialties:**

   - o Enjoy a culinary journey with gut-friendly recipes from different cultures around the world.

7. **Resources and References:**

   - o **Ingredient Guide and Glossary:** Familiarize yourself with essential ingredients and terms.

   - o **Further Reading:** Find additional resources to expand your knowledge.

8. **Conclusion:**

   - o Recap key points and get inspired to maintain your gut health journey long-term.

Making the Recipes Work for You

Each recipe in this cookbook has been carefully crafted to be both delicious and beneficial for your gut. Here's how to get the most out of them:

- **Ingredients:** Pay attention to the ingredients list. Many recipes include ingredients that are specifically chosen for their gut health benefits, such as high-fiber vegetables, fermented foods, and prebiotic-rich items.

- **Instructions:** Follow the step-by-step instructions to ensure you're preparing the dishes correctly. This will help you maximize the health benefits and flavor of each meal.

- **Nutritional Values:** Each recipe includes nutritional information to help you understand the contribution of each dish to your overall diet. This can be particularly useful if you're tracking specific nutrients or adhering to a particular dietary plan.

Tailoring the Cookbook to Your Needs

The "GUT CHECK COOKBOOK" is designed to be flexible and adaptable. Here are some tips to tailor it to your needs:

- **Special Diets:** If you have specific dietary requirements, refer to the Special Diets section for recipes that cater to gluten-free, dairy-free, low-FODMAP, and plant-based diets.

- **Meal Planning:** Use the sample meal plans as a guide to structure your week. You can mix and match recipes from different sections to create a plan that suits your preferences and schedule.

- **Lifestyle Integration:** Incorporate the lifestyle tips provided in the relevant sections to complement your dietary changes. Exercise, stress management, and adequate sleep are all crucial components of a healthy gut.

Embracing the Journey

Embarking on a journey to better gut health is an empowering step towards improving your overall well-being. The "GUT CHECK COOKBOOK" is more than just a collection of recipes; it's a comprehensive guide that supports you every step of the way. By understanding the vital role of your gut, making mindful dietary choices, and adopting healthy lifestyle habits, you can unlock a new level of vitality and health.

Chapter 1: Understanding Your Gut

Your gut, often called the digestive tract or gastrointestinal (GI) tract, is an intricate system that does much more than process food. It begins at the mouth and extends through the esophagus, stomach, small intestine, and large intestine, ending at the rectum and anus. This complex network is responsible for digesting food, absorbing nutrients, and eliminating waste. But its role extends beyond mere digestion; it plays a crucial part in your overall health and well-being.

Anatomy and Function

Your gut, a marvel of biological engineering, is more than just a conduit for food. It is a complex, dynamic system that performs a myriad of functions essential for sustaining life. Let's explore the anatomy and function of this vital system.

1. The Mouth and Esophagus

- **Digestion Begins:** The process of digestion starts in the mouth. Chewing breaks down food into smaller pieces, while saliva, containing enzymes like amylase, begins the chemical breakdown of carbohydrates.

- **Swallowing:** The act of swallowing moves the food from the mouth to the esophagus.

- **The Esophagus:** This muscular tube connects the throat to the stomach. Through rhythmic muscle contractions known as peristalsis, it propels the food downward.

2. The Stomach

- **Storage and Mixing:** The stomach temporarily stores food and mixes it with gastric juices to form chyme, a semi-liquid substance.

- **Chemical Breakdown:** Gastric juices, containing hydrochloric acid and digestive enzymes like pepsin, break down proteins and kill potentially harmful bacteria.

- **Mucosal Protection:** The stomach lining secretes mucus to protect itself from the corrosive effects of gastric acid.

3. The Small Intestine

- **Segments:** The small intestine is divided into three parts: the duodenum, jejunum, and ileum.

- **Duodenum:** Here, chyme is mixed with bile from the liver and digestive enzymes from the pancreas, continuing the chemical breakdown of food.

- **Jejunum and Ileum:** These sections are primarily responsible for nutrient absorption. The inner surface, lined with villi and microvilli, increases the surface area to maximize absorption.

- **Nutrient Absorption:** Nutrients like amino acids, simple sugars, fatty acids, and vitamins are absorbed into the bloodstream through the walls of the small intestine.

4. The Large Intestine

- **Components:** The large intestine includes the cecum, colon, rectum, and anus.

- **Water and Electrolyte Absorption:** The primary function of the large intestine is to absorb water and electrolytes from the remaining indigestible food matter.

- **Formation of Feces:** As water is absorbed, the waste material is compacted into feces. Beneficial bacteria in the colon further break down some of the remaining substances.

- **Waste Elimination:** The rectum stores feces until they are excreted through the anus during a bowel movement.

5. Accessory Organs

- **Liver:** Produces bile, which helps emulsify fats, making them easier to digest.

- **Gallbladder:** Stores and concentrates bile, releasing it into the small intestine as needed.

- **Pancreas:** Produces digestive enzymes and bicarbonate to neutralize stomach acid entering the small intestine. It also secretes insulin and glucagon, hormones that regulate blood sugar levels.

The Gut Microbiome

- **Diverse Ecosystem:** The gut is home to trillions of microorganisms, including bacteria, viruses, fungi, and protozoa, collectively known as the gut microbiome.

- **Microbial Functions:** These microorganisms play crucial roles in digestion, nutrient synthesis, immune function, and even mood regulation.

- **Balance and Health:** A balanced microbiome, with a rich diversity of beneficial bacteria, is essential for maintaining overall health. Dysbiosis, or an imbalance in the microbiome, can lead to various health issues, including digestive disorders, allergies, and mental health conditions.

The Gut-Brain Connection

The gut and brain are intricately connected in a bi-directional communication network known as the gut-brain axis. This connection influences not only digestive health but also mental health, mood, and overall well-being. Understanding the gut-brain connection can help you appreciate the profound impact that your digestive system has on your entire body.

The Vagus Nerve: The Superhighway

- **Primary Pathway:** The vagus nerve is the primary communication pathway between the gut and the brain. This long, wandering nerve extends from the brainstem to various organs, including the heart, lungs, and digestive tract.

- **Neurotransmission:** The vagus nerve transmits signals about the state of the gut to the brain and vice versa. It plays a crucial role in regulating digestive processes, such as enzyme secretion, bile production, and peristalsis (the movement of food through the digestive tract).

Neurotransmitters: Chemical Messengers

- **Serotonin:** Approximately 90% of the body's serotonin, a key neurotransmitter that regulates mood, is produced in the gut. Serotonin influences not only mood but also bowel movements and function.

- **Dopamine:** The gut also produces dopamine, another neurotransmitter associated with pleasure and reward. This highlights the gut's influence on emotions and motivation.

- **Other Neurotransmitters:** The gut produces various other neurotransmitters, such as gamma-aminobutyric acid (GABA), which has a calming effect on the brain and body.

The Microbiome's Role

- **Microbial Influence:** The gut microbiome, the community of trillions of microorganisms living in the digestive tract, plays a pivotal role in the gut-brain connection. These microbes produce metabolites that can affect brain function and behavior.

- **Short-Chain Fatty Acids (SCFAs):** Produced by the fermentation of dietary fibers by gut bacteria, SCFAs like butyrate, propionate, and acetate have been shown to influence brain function and reduce inflammation.

- **Tryptophan Metabolism:** Gut bacteria help metabolize tryptophan, an amino acid precursor to serotonin. This connection underscores how gut health can influence mood and mental health.

Impact on Mental Health

- **Mood Disorders:** Dysbiosis, or an imbalance in the gut microbiome, has been linked to mood disorders such as depression and anxiety. Studies have shown that restoring balance in the gut can alleviate symptoms of these conditions.

- **Stress Response:** Chronic stress can disrupt the gut microbiome, leading to increased permeability of the gut lining (often referred to as "leaky gut") and systemic inflammation, which in turn can affect mental health.

- **Cognitive Function:** Emerging research suggests that gut health can impact cognitive functions such as memory and learning. A healthy gut microbiome is associated with better cognitive performance and a reduced risk of neurodegenerative diseases.

Practical Steps to Support the Gut-Brain Axis

1. **Diet:**

   - **Prebiotics and Probiotics:** Incorporate prebiotic-rich foods (e.g., garlic, onions, bananas) and probiotic foods (e.g., yogurt, kefir, sauerkraut) to support a healthy microbiome.

   - **Fiber:** A diet high in fiber from fruits, vegetables, and whole grains promotes the production of beneficial SCFAs.

   - **Omega-3 Fatty Acids:** Found in fatty fish, flaxseeds, and walnuts, omega-3s support brain health and reduce inflammation.

2. **Lifestyle:**

   - **Stress Management:** Practice stress-reducing activities such as yoga, meditation, and deep breathing exercises to support the gut-brain axis.

   - **Regular Exercise:** Physical activity promotes a healthy gut microbiome and enhances overall brain function.

- o **Adequate Sleep:** Quality sleep is essential for maintaining a healthy gut and supporting cognitive health.

3. **Mindful Eating:**

   - o **Chewing Thoroughly:** Properly chewing food aids digestion and signals the brain about satiety and digestion.

   - o **Eating Slowly:** Taking time to eat allows for better digestion and absorption of nutrients.

Common Issues and Symptoms

Gut health issues can manifest in a variety of ways, affecting not only your digestive system but also your overall health. Identifying these issues early and understanding their symptoms can help you take proactive steps towards better gut health. Here are some common gut health problems and their associated symptoms.

1. Irritable Bowel Syndrome (IBS)

- **Description:** IBS is a chronic condition characterized by abdominal pain and changes in bowel habits without any detectable underlying damage to the digestive tract.

- **Symptoms:**
  - o Abdominal pain or cramping, often relieved by bowel movements
  - o Bloating and gas
  - o Diarrhea, constipation, or alternating between the two
  - o Mucus in the stool

2. Inflammatory Bowel Disease (IBD)

- **Description:** IBD is a group of inflammatory conditions, primarily Crohn's disease and ulcerative colitis, that cause chronic inflammation of the gastrointestinal tract.

- **Symptoms:**
  - o Persistent diarrhea
  - o Abdominal pain and cramping
  - o Blood in the stool
  - o Fatigue and weight loss

o Reduced appetite

3. Small Intestinal Bacterial Overgrowth (SIBO)

- **Description:** SIBO occurs when there is an abnormal increase in the number of bacteria in the small intestine, which can interfere with digestion and nutrient absorption.

- **Symptoms:**

  o Bloating and distension

  o Abdominal pain

  o Diarrhea or constipation

  o Malnutrition and weight loss

  o Fatigue

4. Gastroesophageal Reflux Disease (GERD)

- **Description:** GERD is a chronic condition where stomach acid frequently flows back into the esophagus, causing irritation.

- **Symptoms:**

  o Heartburn, a burning sensation in the chest

  o Regurgitation of food or sour liquid

  o Difficulty swallowing

  o Chronic cough or throat irritation

  o Hoarseness or sore throat

5. Food Intolerances and Allergies

- **Description:** Food intolerances occur when the digestive system is unable to properly break down certain foods, while food allergies involve an immune response to specific food proteins.

- **Symptoms:**

  o Bloating and gas

  o Abdominal pain and cramps

  o Diarrhea or constipation

  o Nausea and vomiting

    o Skin rashes or hives (in the case of allergies)

6. Gut Dysbiosis

- **Description:** Gut dysbiosis refers to an imbalance in the gut microbiome, where harmful bacteria outnumber beneficial bacteria.

- **Symptoms:**

    o Digestive issues like bloating, gas, diarrhea, and constipation

    o Food intolerances

    o Fatigue and brain fog

    o Skin issues like acne, eczema, or rashes

    o Weakened immune function

7. Leaky Gut Syndrome

- **Description:** Leaky gut syndrome, or increased intestinal permeability, occurs when the lining of the small intestine becomes damaged, allowing toxins and undigested food particles to enter the bloodstream.

- **Symptoms:**

    o Chronic diarrhea, constipation, or bloating

    o Nutritional deficiencies

    o Fatigue and headaches

    o Joint pain and widespread inflammation

    o Skin problems, such as eczema or acne

8. Celiac Disease

- **Description:** Celiac disease is an autoimmune disorder where ingestion of gluten leads to damage in the small intestine.

- **Symptoms:**

    o Diarrhea or constipation

    o Abdominal pain and bloating

    o Fatigue

    o Anemia and nutritional deficiencies

    o Dermatitis herpetiformis (a rash associated with celiac disease)

When to Seek Medical Advice

While occasional digestive discomfort is common, persistent or severe symptoms should prompt a visit to a healthcare professional. If you experience any of the following, it's important to seek medical advice:

- Unexplained weight loss

- Severe abdominal pain

- Persistent changes in bowel habits

- Blood in the stool

- Difficulty swallowing

- Symptoms of malnutrition

Chapter 2: The Gut Microbiome

The gut microbiome is a complex and dynamic ecosystem of trillions of microorganisms, including bacteria, viruses, fungi, and other microbes, residing primarily in the intestines. This microbial community plays a crucial role in maintaining overall health and has far-reaching effects on digestion, immunity, and even mental health.

Components of the Gut Microbiome

1. **Bacteria:** The most studied and predominant inhabitants, beneficial bacteria like Lactobacillus and Bifidobacterium are essential for maintaining gut health.

2. **Viruses:** Gut viruses, including bacteriophages, influence bacterial populations and diversity.

3. **Fungi:** Yeasts and other fungi, such as Candida species, are part of the normal gut flora but can cause issues if overgrown.

4. **Other Microbes:** Protozoa and archaea also play roles, though they are less well understood.

Importance of the Gut Microbiome

1. **Digestion and Metabolism:**

   o **Breaking Down Food:** Microbes help break down complex carbohydrates, fibers, and proteins that the human digestive enzymes cannot fully digest.

   o **Fermentation:** The fermentation of dietary fibers by gut bacteria produces short-chain fatty acids (SCFAs) like acetate, propionate, and butyrate, which are beneficial for gut health and energy production.

2. **Nutrient Synthesis:**

   o **Vitamin Production:** Gut bacteria synthesize essential vitamins such as vitamin K and some B vitamins (B12, folate, riboflavin).

   o **Amino Acids:** They also help produce amino acids and other bioactive compounds.

3. **Immune System Support:**

   - **Barrier Function:** A healthy gut microbiome strengthens the intestinal barrier, preventing harmful pathogens from entering the bloodstream.

   - **Immune Modulation:** Gut microbes educate and regulate the immune system, helping to distinguish between harmful and harmless entities.

4. **Mental Health:**

   - **Neurotransmitter Production:** Gut bacteria produce neurotransmitters like serotonin and GABA, which influence mood and cognitive function.

   - **Gut-Brain Axis:** The gut microbiome communicates with the brain through the vagus nerve and other biochemical pathways, impacting stress response, anxiety, and depression.

Factors Influencing the Gut Microbiome

1. **Diet:**

   - **Diverse and Balanced Diet:** Consuming a variety of whole foods, particularly fiber-rich fruits, vegetables, and whole grains, supports a diverse microbiome.

   - **Fermented Foods:** Foods like yogurt, kefir, sauerkraut, and kimchi introduce beneficial probiotics to the gut.

   - **Prebiotics:** These non-digestible fibers found in foods like garlic, onions, and bananas feed beneficial bacteria.

2. **Antibiotics and Medications:**

   - **Antibiotics:** While they kill harmful bacteria, antibiotics also disrupt beneficial gut bacteria, potentially leading to dysbiosis.

   - **Other Medications:** Nonsteroidal anti-inflammatory drugs (NSAIDs) and proton pump inhibitors (PPIs) can also impact gut health.

3. **Lifestyle Factors:**

   - **Stress:** Chronic stress negatively affects the gut microbiome, promoting the growth of harmful bacteria.

   - **Sleep:** Adequate and quality sleep supports a healthy microbiome.

   - **Exercise:** Regular physical activity promotes microbial diversity and gut health.

4. **Environmental Factors:**

   o **Hygiene Hypothesis:** Excessive cleanliness and lack of exposure to diverse microbes in early life may contribute to less robust microbiomes.

   o **Geography and Lifestyle:** Differences in diet, lifestyle, and environmental exposures lead to variations in microbiome composition among populations.

Achieving and Maintaining Gut Balance

A balanced gut microbiome, where beneficial bacteria thrive and outnumber harmful ones, is crucial for overall health. The benefits of maintaining this balance extend far beyond digestion, impacting numerous aspects of physical and mental well-being.

1. Improved Digestion and Nutrient Absorption

- **Efficient Digestion:** A balanced gut microbiome aids in the breakdown of complex carbohydrates, proteins, and fats, making digestion more efficient.

- **Enhanced Nutrient Absorption:** Beneficial bacteria help increase the bioavailability of nutrients, ensuring that your body absorbs essential vitamins, minerals, and amino acids effectively.

- **Reduced Digestive Discomfort:** Balance in the gut microbiome reduces common digestive issues such as bloating, gas, constipation, and diarrhea.

2. Strengthened Immune System

- **Barrier Function:** A healthy gut microbiome supports the integrity of the intestinal lining, preventing harmful pathogens and toxins from entering the bloodstream.

- **Immune Regulation:** Beneficial bacteria help regulate the immune system, enhancing its ability to respond to infections and reducing the risk of autoimmune conditions.

- **Inflammation Control:** A balanced microbiome reduces chronic inflammation, which is linked to many diseases, including inflammatory bowel disease (IBD), arthritis, and cardiovascular disease.

3. Enhanced Mental Health

- **Mood Regulation:** The gut microbiome produces neurotransmitters like serotonin and dopamine, which play a crucial role in regulating mood and preventing depression and anxiety.

- **Stress Reduction:** A balanced gut microbiome helps modulate the body's stress response, reducing the impact of chronic stress on mental health.

- **Cognitive Function:** Emerging research suggests that a healthy gut microbiome supports cognitive functions such as memory, learning, and focus.

4. Weight Management and Metabolic Health

- **Appetite Regulation:** Gut bacteria influence the production of hormones that regulate appetite, such as leptin and ghrelin, helping to maintain a healthy weight.

- **Metabolic Efficiency:** A balanced microbiome enhances metabolic processes, improving energy expenditure and reducing the risk of metabolic disorders like obesity and type 2 diabetes.

- **Fat Storage:** Beneficial bacteria can influence the way your body stores fat and regulates blood sugar levels.

5. Skin Health

- **Reduced Inflammation:** A healthy gut reduces systemic inflammation, which can lead to clearer skin and reduced symptoms of conditions like acne, eczema, and psoriasis.

- **Nutrient Delivery:** Enhanced nutrient absorption ensures that the skin receives essential vitamins and minerals necessary for repair and regeneration.

6. Better Sleep Quality

- **Sleep Regulation:** The gut microbiome influences the production of neurotransmitters and hormones that regulate sleep cycles, such as melatonin.

- **Stress Management:** By reducing stress and anxiety, a balanced microbiome contributes to more restful and uninterrupted sleep.

7. Longevity and Disease Prevention

- **Chronic Disease Risk Reduction:** A healthy gut microbiome is linked to a lower risk of chronic diseases, including cardiovascular disease, type 2 diabetes, and certain cancers.

- **Healthy Aging:** Maintaining a balanced gut microbiome supports healthy aging by preserving cognitive function, immune response, and metabolic health.

Practical Tips for Maintaining Gut Balance

1. **Diet:**

   o **Diverse and Fiber-Rich Diet:** Eat a wide variety of plant-based foods rich in fiber to nourish beneficial bacteria.

   o **Fermented Foods:** Include probiotic-rich foods like yogurt, kefir, sauerkraut, and kimchi in your diet.

   o **Limit Processed Foods:** Reduce intake of processed foods, sugar, and artificial sweeteners, which can disrupt the microbiome balance.

2. **Lifestyle:**

   o **Regular Exercise:** Engage in regular physical activity to promote gut health and microbial diversity.

   o **Stress Management:** Practice stress-reducing techniques such as mindfulness, meditation, and deep breathing exercises.

   o **Adequate Sleep:** Ensure you get enough quality sleep to support overall health and gut function.

3. **Probiotics and Supplements:**

   o **Probiotic Supplements:** Consider taking high-quality probiotic supplements, especially after antibiotic use, to restore gut balance.

   o **Prebiotic Supplements:** If dietary intake is insufficient, supplements like inulin or psyllium husk can help support gut health.

The Cornerstone of Gut Health

Diet is the cornerstone of gut health, playing a vital role in shaping the gut microbiome and influencing overall well-being. What you eat directly affects the diversity and abundance of gut bacteria, which in turn impacts digestion, immunity, mental health, and disease prevention.

Key Functions of Diet in Gut Health

1. **Nourishing Beneficial Bacteria**

   o **Prebiotics:** Dietary fibers found in foods such as garlic, onions, leeks, bananas, and asparagus act as prebiotics, feeding beneficial gut bacteria and promoting their growth.

   o **Probiotics:** Fermented foods like yogurt, kefir, sauerkraut, kimchi, and miso introduce live beneficial bacteria into the gut, enhancing microbial diversity and balance.

2. **Maintaining Gut Lining Integrity**

   o **Healthy Fats:** Omega-3 fatty acids, found in fatty fish, flaxseeds, and walnuts, help maintain the integrity of the gut lining and reduce inflammation.

   o **Amino Acids:** Proteins from lean meats, legumes, and eggs provide essential amino acids like glutamine, which support the repair and maintenance of the gut lining.

3. **Regulating Immune Function**

   o **Vitamins and Minerals:** A diet rich in vitamins (A, C, D, E) and minerals (zinc, selenium) supports the immune system, enhancing its ability to respond to infections and maintain gut health.

   o **Antioxidants:** Polyphenols and other antioxidants found in fruits, vegetables, nuts, and seeds help reduce oxidative stress and inflammation in the gut.

4. **Supporting Digestion and Nutrient Absorption**

   o **Fiber:** Insoluble and soluble fibers aid in digestion and the absorption of nutrients, ensuring that the body receives essential vitamins and minerals.

   o **Enzymes:** Certain foods, like pineapples and papayas, contain natural digestive enzymes that assist in breaking down proteins and other nutrients for better absorption.

5. **Balancing Gut Microbiome**

   o **Diverse Diet:** Consuming a variety of whole foods, particularly plant-based ones, ensures a diverse gut microbiome, which is associated with better health outcomes.

   o **Limiting Harmful Foods:** Reducing the intake of processed foods, refined sugars, and artificial sweeteners helps prevent the overgrowth of harmful bacteria and yeast.

Impact of Specific Dietary Choices on Gut Health

1. **High-Fiber Foods**

   o **Benefits:** Fiber-rich foods like fruits, vegetables, whole grains, and legumes promote regular bowel movements, feed beneficial bacteria, and reduce the risk of digestive disorders.

   o **Examples:** Apples, carrots, brown rice, lentils, and beans.

2. **Fermented Foods**

   o **Benefits:** Fermented foods introduce probiotics that enhance gut flora, improve digestion, and boost the immune system.

   o **Examples:** Yogurt, kefir, kimchi, sauerkraut, and miso.

3. **Healthy Fats**

   o **Benefits:** Omega-3 fatty acids and other healthy fats reduce inflammation, support the gut lining, and contribute to a balanced microbiome.

   o **Examples:** Salmon, chia seeds, flaxseeds, and olive oil.

4. **Polyphenol-Rich Foods**

   o **Benefits:** Polyphenols have antioxidant properties that support gut health by reducing inflammation and supporting beneficial bacteria.

   o **Examples:** Dark chocolate, berries, green tea, and red wine.

5. **Prebiotic Foods**

   o **Benefits:** Prebiotics, found in foods like garlic, onions, and asparagus, nourish beneficial gut bacteria, promoting a healthy and balanced microbiome.

   o **Examples:** Garlic, onions, leeks, bananas, and asparagus.

Foods to Limit or Avoid for Optimal Gut Health

1. **Processed Foods**

   o **Impact:** High in unhealthy fats, sugars, and additives, processed foods can disrupt the gut microbiome and promote inflammation.

   o **Examples:** Fast food, packaged snacks, and sugary cereals.

2. **Refined Sugars**

   o **Impact:** Excessive sugar intake can feed harmful bacteria and yeast, leading to an imbalance in the gut microbiome.

   o **Examples:** Candy, pastries, and soda.

3. **Artificial Sweeteners**

   o **Impact:** Some artificial sweeteners may negatively affect gut bacteria and contribute to dysbiosis.

   o **Examples:** Aspartame, sucralose, and saccharin.

4. **Red and Processed Meats**

   o **Impact:** High consumption of red and processed meats is linked to an increased risk of colorectal cancer and may promote the growth of harmful gut bacteria.

   o **Examples:** Bacon, sausages, hot dogs, and deli meats.

Practical Dietary Strategies for a Healthy Gut

1. **Eat a Diverse Diet:**

   o Incorporate a wide variety of fruits, vegetables, whole grains, legumes, nuts, and seeds to ensure a diverse intake of nutrients and fibers.

2. **Include Fermented Foods:**

   o Regularly consume fermented foods to introduce beneficial probiotics into your diet.

3. **Stay Hydrated:**

   o Drink plenty of water throughout the day to aid digestion and maintain a healthy gut lining.

4. **Limit Processed and Sugary Foods:**

   o   Reduce intake of processed foods, refined sugars, and artificial sweeteners to avoid disrupting the gut microbiome.

5. **Balanced Meals:**

   o   Ensure your meals include a balance of fiber, protein, and healthy fats to support overall digestive health.

Chapter 3: Diet in Gut Health

Diet is the cornerstone of gut health, playing a vital role in shaping the gut microbiome and influencing overall well-being. What you eat directly affects the diversity and abundance of gut bacteria, which in turn impacts digestion, immunity, mental health, and disease prevention.

Key Functions of Diet in Gut Health

1. **Nourishing Beneficial Bacteria**

   - **Prebiotics:** Dietary fibers found in foods such as garlic, onions, leeks, bananas, and asparagus act as prebiotics, feeding beneficial gut bacteria and promoting their growth.

   - **Probiotics:** Fermented foods like yogurt, kefir, sauerkraut, kimchi, and miso introduce live beneficial bacteria into the gut, enhancing microbial diversity and balance.

2. **Maintaining Gut Lining Integrity**

   - **Healthy Fats:** Omega-3 fatty acids, found in fatty fish, flaxseeds, and walnuts, help maintain the integrity of the gut lining and reduce inflammation.

   - **Amino Acids:** Proteins from lean meats, legumes, and eggs provide essential amino acids like glutamine, which support the repair and maintenance of the gut lining.

3. **Regulating Immune Function**

   - **Vitamins and Minerals:** A diet rich in vitamins (A, C, D, E) and minerals (zinc, selenium) supports the immune system, enhancing its ability to respond to infections and maintain gut health.

   - **Antioxidants:** Polyphenols and other antioxidants found in fruits, vegetables, nuts, and seeds help reduce oxidative stress and inflammation in the gut.

4. **Supporting Digestion and Nutrient Absorption**

   - **Fiber:** Insoluble and soluble fibers aid in digestion and the absorption of nutrients, ensuring that the body receives essential vitamins and minerals.

   - **Enzymes:** Certain foods, like pineapples and papayas, contain natural digestive enzymes that assist in breaking down proteins and other nutrients for better absorption.

5. **Balancing Gut Microbiome**

   o **Diverse Diet:** Consuming a variety of whole foods, particularly plant-based ones, ensures a diverse gut microbiome, which is associated with better health outcomes.

   o **Limiting Harmful Foods:** Reducing the intake of processed foods, refined sugars, and artificial sweeteners helps prevent the overgrowth of harmful bacteria and yeast.

Impact of Specific Dietary Choices on Gut Health

1. **High-Fiber Foods**

   o **Benefits:** Fiber-rich foods like fruits, vegetables, whole grains, and legumes promote regular bowel movements, feed beneficial bacteria, and reduce the risk of digestive disorders.

   o **Examples:** Apples, carrots, brown rice, lentils, and beans.

2. **Fermented Foods**

   o **Benefits:** Fermented foods introduce probiotics that enhance gut flora, improve digestion, and boost the immune system.

   o **Examples:** Yogurt, kefir, kimchi, sauerkraut, and miso.

3. **Healthy Fats**

   o **Benefits:** Omega-3 fatty acids and other healthy fats reduce inflammation, support the gut lining, and contribute to a balanced microbiome.

   o **Examples:** Salmon, chia seeds, flaxseeds, and olive oil.

4. **Polyphenol-Rich Foods**

   o **Benefits:** Polyphenols have antioxidant properties that support gut health by reducing inflammation and supporting beneficial bacteria.

   o **Examples:** Dark chocolate, berries, green tea, and red wine.

5. **Prebiotic Foods**

   o **Benefits:** Prebiotics, found in foods like garlic, onions, and asparagus, nourish beneficial gut bacteria, promoting a healthy and balanced microbiome.

   o **Examples:** Garlic, onions, leeks, bananas, and asparagus.

Foods to Promote for Gut Health

Promoting the right foods can significantly enhance gut health, fostering a diverse and balanced microbiome, supporting digestion, and bolstering the immune system. Here are key foods to include in your diet:

1. **Fiber-Rich Foods**

   o **Whole Grains:** Brown rice, quinoa, oats, barley, and whole wheat products.

      ▪ *Benefits:* These grains provide insoluble and soluble fibers that aid digestion and promote regular bowel movements.

   o **Fruits:** Apples, bananas, berries, oranges, and pears.

      ▪ *Benefits:* Fruits are rich in vitamins, antioxidants, and dietary fibers that support gut bacteria.

   o **Vegetables:** Broccoli, carrots, Brussels sprouts, spinach, and sweet potatoes.

      ▪ *Benefits:* Vegetables provide essential fibers, vitamins, and minerals that nourish the gut microbiome.

   o **Legumes:** Beans, lentils, chickpeas, and peas.

      ▪ *Benefits:* Legumes are excellent sources of fiber and protein that feed beneficial gut bacteria.

2. **Prebiotic Foods**

   o **Garlic, Onions, and Leeks:** Rich in inulin, a type of prebiotic fiber.

      ▪ *Benefits:* These foods help stimulate the growth of beneficial gut bacteria.

   o **Asparagus and Jerusalem Artichokes:** High in prebiotic fibers.

      ▪ *Benefits:* They support a healthy and balanced gut microbiome.

3. **Probiotic Foods**

   o **Yogurt and Kefir:** Contain live beneficial bacteria.

      ▪ *Benefits:* These dairy products introduce probiotics that enhance microbial diversity and gut health.

- **Sauerkraut and Kimchi:** Fermented vegetables rich in probiotics.
    - *Benefits:* These foods support digestion and boost the immune system.
- **Miso and Tempeh:** Fermented soy products.
    - *Benefits:* They provide probiotics and support gut microbiome balance.

4. **Polyphenol-Rich Foods**

- **Dark Chocolate and Cocoa:** Rich in polyphenols.
    - *Benefits:* Polyphenols have antioxidant properties that support beneficial gut bacteria.
- **Berries:** Blueberries, strawberries, raspberries, and blackberries.
    - *Benefits:* These fruits provide antioxidants that reduce inflammation and support gut health.
- **Green Tea and Red Wine:** Contain high levels of polyphenols.
    - *Benefits:* These beverages support gut health by promoting beneficial bacteria growth.

5. **Healthy Fats**

- **Fatty Fish:** Salmon, mackerel, and sardines.
    - *Benefits:* Rich in omega-3 fatty acids, these fish reduce inflammation and support the gut lining.
- **Nuts and Seeds:** Almonds, walnuts, chia seeds, and flaxseeds.
    - *Benefits:* Provide healthy fats, fiber, and polyphenols that promote gut health.
- **Olive Oil:** Extra virgin olive oil.
    - *Benefits:* Contains healthy fats and polyphenols that support gut microbiome balance.

Foods to Avoid for Gut Health

Avoiding certain foods can prevent disruptions in the gut microbiome and reduce inflammation, promoting overall digestive health. Here are key foods to limit or avoid:

1. **Processed Foods**
   - **Examples:** Fast food, packaged snacks, and sugary cereals.
     - *Impact:* High in unhealthy fats, sugars, and additives, processed foods can disrupt the gut microbiome and promote inflammation.

2. **Refined Sugars**
   - **Examples:** Candy, pastries, and soda.
     - *Impact:* Excessive sugar intake can feed harmful bacteria and yeast, leading to an imbalance in the gut microbiome.

3. **Artificial Sweeteners**
   - **Examples:** Aspartame, sucralose, and saccharin.
     - *Impact:* Some artificial sweeteners may negatively affect gut bacteria and contribute to dysbiosis.

4. **Red and Processed Meats**
   - **Examples:** Bacon, sausages, hot dogs, and deli meats.
     - *Impact:* High consumption of red and processed meats is linked to an increased risk of colorectal cancer and may promote the growth of harmful gut bacteria.

5. **High-Fat and Fried Foods**
   - **Examples:** Fried chicken, French fries, and potato chips.
     - *Impact:* These foods can slow digestion, cause discomfort, and contribute to an imbalance in the gut microbiome.

6. **Excessive Alcohol**
   - **Impact:** Overconsumption of alcohol can disrupt the gut lining and microbiome, leading to inflammation and digestive issues.

Practical Tips for a Gut-Friendly Diet

1. **Eat a Diverse Diet:**

   o Incorporate a wide variety of fruits, vegetables, whole grains, legumes, nuts, and seeds to ensure a diverse intake of nutrients and fibers.

2. **Include Fermented Foods:**

   o Regularly consume fermented foods to introduce beneficial probiotics into your diet.

3. **Stay Hydrated:**

   o Drink plenty of water throughout the day to aid digestion and maintain a healthy gut lining.

4. **Limit Processed and Sugary Foods:**

   o Reduce intake of processed foods, refined sugars, and artificial sweeteners to avoid disrupting the gut microbiome.

5. **Balanced Meals:**

   o Ensure your meals include a balance of fiber, protein, and healthy fats to support overall digestive health.

Probiotics and Prebiotics

Understanding Probiotics

Probiotics are live microorganisms, often referred to as "good" or "friendly" bacteria, that provide numerous health benefits when consumed in adequate amounts. These beneficial bacteria help maintain a healthy balance in the gut microbiome, support digestion, enhance immune function, and may even improve mental health.

Sources of Probiotics:

1. **Yogurt:** Contains live cultures such as Lactobacillus and Bifidobacterium.

   o *Benefits:* Enhances digestion, boosts the immune system, and can improve lactose intolerance.

2. **Kefir:** A fermented milk drink rich in probiotics.

   o *Benefits:* Supports gut health, aids digestion, and can help combat gut inflammation.

3. **Sauerkraut:** Fermented cabbage rich in Lactobacillus bacteria.

   o *Benefits:* Supports digestive health, provides vitamins C and K, and has anti-inflammatory properties.

4. **Kimchi:** A spicy Korean fermented vegetable dish.

   o *Benefits:* Promotes a healthy gut, boosts immunity, and supports cardiovascular health.

5. **Miso:** A traditional Japanese fermented soybean paste.

   o *Benefits:* Provides probiotics, supports digestion, and is rich in essential minerals.

6. **Tempeh:** A fermented soybean product.

   o *Benefits:* Contains probiotics, is a good source of protein, and provides B vitamins.

7. **Kombucha:** A fermented tea drink.

   o *Benefits:* Rich in probiotics, helps detoxify the body, and supports digestive health.

8. **Pickles:** Fermented cucumbers.

   o *Benefits:* Contain probiotics, support digestion, and provide antioxidants.

Understanding Prebiotics

Prebiotics are non-digestible fibers that serve as food for probiotics, helping them thrive in the gut. They play a crucial role in maintaining a healthy gut microbiome by promoting the growth and activity of beneficial bacteria.

Sources of Prebiotics:

1. **Garlic:** Contains inulin, a type of prebiotic fiber.

   o *Benefits:* Supports the growth of beneficial bacteria, enhances immune function, and has anti-inflammatory properties.

2. **Onions:** Rich in inulin and fructooligosaccharides (FOS).

   o *Benefits:* Promote gut health, support digestion, and provide antioxidants.

3. **Leeks:** High in inulin and FOS.

   o *Benefits:* Support beneficial bacteria, aid digestion, and are rich in vitamins A and K.

4. **Asparagus:** Contains inulin.

   o *Benefits:* Supports gut health, aids digestion, and provides vitamins and minerals.

5. **Bananas:** Provide resistant starch and FOS.

   o *Benefits:* Promote healthy gut bacteria, aid digestion, and provide essential nutrients.

6. **Jerusalem Artichokes:** Rich in inulin.

   o *Benefits:* Support beneficial bacteria, improve digestion, and are a good source of iron.

7. **Chicory Root:** Contains high levels of inulin.

   o *Benefits:* Supports gut health, aids digestion, and can help regulate blood sugar levels.

8. **Barley:** Provides beta-glucan and other prebiotic fibers.

   o *Benefits:* Supports gut health, reduces cholesterol levels, and aids digestion.

9. **Oats:** Rich in beta-glucan.

   o *Benefits:* Promote beneficial bacteria, support digestion, and help regulate blood sugar levels.

10. **Apples:** Contain pectin, a type of prebiotic fiber.

   o *Benefits:* Support gut health, aid digestion, and provide antioxidants.

Benefits of Combining Probiotics and Prebiotics

Combining probiotics and prebiotics, known as synbiotics, can enhance the beneficial effects on gut health by ensuring that the probiotics have the necessary food to thrive. This synergy promotes a balanced and diverse gut microbiome, which is essential for optimal digestive health, immune function, and overall well-being.

Health Benefits of Probiotics and Prebiotics:

1. **Enhanced Digestive Health:**

   o Probiotics help break down food, produce essential vitamins, and support nutrient absorption.

   o Prebiotics feed beneficial bacteria, promoting a healthy gut environment and regular bowel movements.

2. **Improved Immune Function:**

   o Probiotics enhance the body's immune response by increasing the production of antibodies and supporting the gut barrier.

   o Prebiotics stimulate the growth of beneficial bacteria, which can outcompete harmful pathogens and support immune health.

3. **Reduced Inflammation:**

   o Probiotics can help reduce inflammation in the gut and throughout the body by modulating the immune response.

   o Prebiotics support the growth of anti-inflammatory bacteria, contributing to overall health.

4. **Better Mental Health:**

   o The gut-brain axis allows probiotics to influence brain function and mental health by producing neurotransmitters such as serotonin.

   o Prebiotics can support this process by promoting a healthy gut environment.

Enhanced Nutrient Absorption:

- o Probiotics aid in the digestion and absorption of nutrients, ensuring that the body receives essential vitamins and minerals.

- o Prebiotics support the growth of bacteria that produce short-chain fatty acids (SCFAs), which are important for nutrient absorption.

Practical Tips for Incorporating Probiotics and Prebiotics

1. **Diverse Diet:**

   - o Incorporate a variety of probiotic and prebiotic-rich foods into your diet to ensure a diverse and balanced gut microbiome.

2. **Regular Consumption:**

   - o Regularly consume fermented foods and prebiotic-rich foods to maintain a healthy balance of gut bacteria.

3. **Probiotic Supplements:**

   - o Consider taking high-quality probiotic supplements, especially after antibiotic use, to replenish beneficial bacteria.

4. **Prebiotic Supplements:**

   - o If dietary intake is insufficient, consider using prebiotic supplements like inulin or psyllium husk to feed beneficial gut bacteria.

5. **Mindful Eating:**

   - o Eat a balanced diet, avoid excessive consumption of processed foods, and stay hydrated to support overall gut health.

Chapter 4: Breakfasts Recipes

Smoothie with Spinach and Berries

Prep Time: 5 minutes | **Cook Time:** 0 minutes | **Per Serving:** 1 serving

Ingredients:

- 1 cup spinach leaves (fresh or frozen)
- 1/2 cup mixed berries (strawberries, blueberries)
- 1/2 banana, sliced
- 1 tablespoon chia seeds
- 1 cup unsweetened almond milk
- Ice cubes (optional)

Instructions:

1. Combine spinach, mixed berries, banana, chia seeds, and almond milk in a blender.
2. Blend until smooth and creamy.
3. Add ice cubes if desired and blend again.
4. Pour into a glass and enjoy the refreshing Smoothie with Spinach and Berries.

Nutritional Value (Approx.): Calories: 150 | Protein: 5g | Fiber: 8g | Healthy Fats: 5g | Carbohydrates: 20g

Chia Seed Pudding

Prep Time: 5 minutes (+ refrigeration) | **Cook Time:** 0 minutes | **Per Serving:** 1 serving

Ingredients:

- 1/4 cup chia seeds
- 1 cup unsweetened almond milk
- 1/2 teaspoon vanilla extract
- 1 tablespoon honey or maple syrup (optional)
- Fresh fruit (berries, mango) for topping

Instructions:

1. In a bowl, mix chia seeds, almond milk, vanilla extract, and honey (if using).

2. Stir well to combine. Cover and refrigerate overnight or for at least 4 hours until it thickens.

3. Stir again before serving. Top with fresh fruit and enjoy the nutritious Chia Seed Pudding.

Nutritional Value (Approx.): Calories: 180 | Protein: 6g | Fiber: 10g | Healthy Fats: 9g | Carbohydrates: 20g

Avocado Toast

Prep Time: 5 minutes | **Cook Time:** 0 minutes | **Per Serving:** 1 serving

Ingredients:

- 1 ripe avocado
- 2 slices whole grain bread, toasted
- 1/2 lemon, juiced
- Cherry tomatoes, sliced
- Olive oil, for drizzling
- Salt and pepper, to taste

Instructions:

1. Mash the avocado in a bowl and mix with lemon juice, salt, and pepper.
2. Spread the mashed avocado evenly on toasted bread slices.
3. Top with sliced cherry tomatoes.
4. Drizzle with olive oil and season with additional salt and pepper if desired.
5. Serve immediately and enjoy the delicious Avocado Toast.

Nutritional Value (Approx.): Calories: 300 | Protein: 7g | Fiber: 10g | Healthy Fats: 15g | Carbohydrates: 30g

Greek Yogurt Parfait

Prep Time: 5 minutes | **Cook Time:** 0 minutes | **Per Serving:** 1 serving

Ingredients:

- 1 cup Greek yogurt
- 1 tablespoon honey or maple syrup (optional)
- 1/4 cup granola
- Mixed berries (raspberries, blueberries)
- Almonds, sliced

Instructions:

1. In a glass or bowl, layer Greek yogurt with honey (if using), granola, and mixed berries.
2. Repeat layers as desired.
3. Top with sliced almonds.
4. Serve chilled and enjoy the creamy and nutritious Greek Yogurt Parfait.

Nutritional Value (Approx.): Calories: 250 | Protein: 15g | Fiber: 5g | Healthy Fats: 8g | Carbohydrates: 30g

Oatmeal with Berries and Almonds

Prep Time: 5 minutes | **Cook Time:** 10 minutes | **Per Serving:** 1 serving

Ingredients:

- 1/2 cup rolled oats
- 1 cup almond milk (or any milk of choice)
- 1/2 cup mixed berries (strawberries, raspberries, blueberries)
- 1 tablespoon almonds, sliced
- 1 tablespoon honey or maple syrup (optional)

Instructions:

1. In a small saucepan, bring almond milk to a boil.
2. Stir in rolled oats and reduce heat to low.
3. Cook for about 5-7 minutes, stirring occasionally, until oats are tender and creamy.
4. Remove from heat and stir in mixed berries.
5. Transfer to a bowl and top with sliced almonds.
6. Drizzle with honey or maple syrup if desired.
7. Serve warm and enjoy the hearty Oatmeal with Berries and Almonds.

Nutritional Value (Approx.): Calories: 300 | Protein: 8g | Fiber: 7g | Healthy Fats: 7g | Carbohydrates: 50g

Quinoa Breakfast Bowl

Prep Time: 10 minutes | **Cook Time:** 15 minutes | **Per Serving:** 1 serving

Ingredients:

- 1/2 cup quinoa, rinsed
- 1 cup water or vegetable broth
- 1/2 avocado, sliced
- 1 egg, boiled or poached
- Handful of spinach leaves
- Cherry tomatoes, halved
- Salt and pepper, to taste

Instructions:

1. In a saucepan, bring water or vegetable broth to a boil.
2. Add quinoa, reduce heat to low, cover, and simmer for about 15 minutes or until quinoa is tender and water is absorbed.
3. Fluff quinoa with a fork and transfer to a bowl.
4. Top with sliced avocado, boiled or poached egg, spinach leaves, and cherry tomatoes.
5. Season with salt and pepper to taste.
6. Serve warm and enjoy the nutritious Quinoa Breakfast Bowl.

Nutritional Value (Approx.): Calories: 350 | Protein: 15g | Fiber: 8g | Healthy Fats: 15g | Carbohydrates: 40g

Blueberry Buckwheat Pancakes

Prep Time: 10 minutes | **Cook Time:** 10 minutes | **Per Serving:** Makes 4 pancakes

Ingredients:

- 1 cup buckwheat flour
- 1 teaspoon baking powder
- 1/2 teaspoon baking soda
- 1/4 teaspoon salt
- 1 cup almond milk (or any milk of choice)
- 1 egg
- 1 tablespoon honey or maple syrup
- 1/2 cup blueberries (fresh or frozen)
- Coconut oil or butter for cooking

Instructions:

1. In a bowl, whisk together buckwheat flour, baking powder, baking soda, and salt.
2. In another bowl, whisk almond milk, egg, and honey or maple syrup.
3. Pour wet ingredients into dry ingredients and stir until just combined.
4. Gently fold in blueberries.
5. Heat coconut oil or butter in a skillet over medium heat.
6. Pour 1/4 cup of batter onto the skillet for each pancake.
7. Cook until bubbles form on the surface, then flip and cook until golden brown.
8. Repeat with remaining batter.
9. Serve warm and enjoy the fluffy Blueberry Buckwheat Pancakes.

Nutritional Value (Approx. per pancake): Calories: 150 | Protein: 5g | Fiber: 3g | Healthy Fats: 3g | Carbohydrates: 25g

Spinach and Mushroom Egg White Omelette

Prep Time: 5 minutes | **Cook Time:** 10 minutes | **Per Serving:** 1 serving

Ingredients:

- 3 egg whites
- Handful of spinach leaves
- 1/2 cup mushrooms, sliced
- 1 tablespoon olive oil
- Salt and pepper, to taste

Instructions:

1. In a bowl, whisk egg whites until frothy.
2. Heat olive oil in a non-stick skillet over medium heat.
3. Add mushrooms and sauté until tender.
4. Add spinach leaves and cook until wilted.
5. Pour egg whites over the vegetables in the skillet.
6. Season with salt and pepper.
7. Cook until edges set, then gently lift edges and tilt skillet to let uncooked egg flow to the edges.
8. Fold omelette in half and cook for another minute until cooked through.
9. Slide onto a plate and serve hot.
10. Enjoy the healthy and protein-packed Spinach and Mushroom Egg White Omelette.

Nutritional Value (Approx.): Calories: 150 | Protein: 15g | Fiber: 3g | Healthy Fats: 7g | Carbohydrates: 5g

Chapter 5: Lunch Recipes

Grilled Chicken Salad with Mixed Greens

Prep Time: 15 minutes | **Cook Time:** 15 minutes | **Per Serving:** 1 serving

Ingredients:

- 4 oz chicken breast, grilled and sliced
- Mixed greens (spinach, arugula, lettuce)
- Cherry tomatoes, halved
- Cucumber, sliced
- Red onion, thinly sliced
- Avocado, sliced
- Olive oil
- Balsamic vinegar or lemon juice
- Salt and pepper, to taste

Instructions:

1. Season chicken breast with salt and pepper, then grill until fully cooked. Slice thinly.
2. In a large bowl, combine mixed greens, cherry tomatoes, cucumber, red onion, and avocado.
3. Drizzle with olive oil and balsamic vinegar or lemon juice.
4. Add grilled chicken slices on top.
5. Toss gently to combine.
6. Serve immediately and enjoy the fresh and nutritious Grilled Chicken Salad with Mixed Greens.

Nutritional Value (Approx.): Calories: 350 | Protein: 30g | Fiber: 8g | Healthy Fats: 15g | Carbohydrates: 20g

Quinoa and Black Bean Stuffed Bell Peppers

Prep Time: 15 minutes | **Cook Time:** 30 minutes | **Per Serving:** 1 serving

Ingredients:

- 2 bell peppers, halved and seeded
- 1/2 cup quinoa, cooked
- 1/2 cup black beans, cooked
- 1/2 cup corn kernels (fresh or frozen)
- 1/4 cup salsa
- 1/2 teaspoon cumin
- Salt and pepper, to taste
- Fresh cilantro, chopped (optional)

Instructions:

1. Preheat oven to 375°F (190°C).
2. In a bowl, mix cooked quinoa, black beans, corn kernels, salsa, cumin, salt, and pepper.
3. Spoon quinoa mixture into each bell pepper half.
4. Place stuffed bell peppers on a baking sheet lined with parchment paper.
5. Bake for 25-30 minutes until peppers are tender.
6. Remove from oven and sprinkle with chopped cilantro if desired.
7. Serve warm and enjoy the flavorful Quinoa and Black Bean Stuffed Bell Peppers.

Nutritional Value (Approx. per serving, 1 stuffed pepper): Calories: 250 | Protein: 10g | Fiber: 10g | Healthy Fats: 3g | Carbohydrates: 45g

Lentil Soup with Kale and Carrots

Prep Time: 10 minutes | **Cook Time:** 30 minutes | **Per Serving:** 1 serving

Ingredients:

- 1 cup lentils, rinsed
- 4 cups vegetable broth
- 1 onion, chopped
- 2 carrots, diced
- 2 cups kale, chopped
- 2 cloves garlic, minced
- 1 teaspoon dried thyme
- Salt and pepper, to taste
- Olive oil

Instructions:

1. Heat olive oil in a large pot over medium heat.
2. Add chopped onion and carrots, sauté until softened.
3. Stir in minced garlic and dried thyme, cook for 1 minute until fragrant.
4. Add rinsed lentils and vegetable broth.
5. Bring to a boil, then reduce heat to low and simmer for 20-25 minutes until lentils are tender.
6. Stir in chopped kale and cook for an additional 5 minutes until kale is wilted.
7. Season with salt and pepper to taste.
8. Serve hot and enjoy the hearty Lentil Soup with Kale and Carrots.

Nutritional Value (Approx. per serving): Calories: 300 | Protein: 15g | Fiber: 15g | Healthy Fats: 5g | Carbohydrates: 50g

Salmon and Avocado Wrap with Whole Grain Tortilla

Prep Time: 10 minutes | **Cook Time:** 10 minutes | **Per Serving:** 1 serving

Ingredients:

- 4 oz salmon fillet
- 1 whole grain tortilla
- 1/2 avocado, sliced
- Mixed greens (spinach, lettuce)
- Tomato, sliced
- Greek yogurt or mayo (optional)
- Lemon wedges
- Salt and pepper, to taste

Instructions:

1. Season salmon fillet with salt and pepper.
2. Grill or bake salmon until cooked through, about 5-7 minutes per side.
3. Warm whole grain tortilla in a skillet or microwave.
4. Spread Greek yogurt or mayo (if using) on tortilla.
5. Layer with mixed greens, sliced avocado, tomato slices, and grilled salmon.
6. Squeeze lemon juice over the ingredients.
7. Roll up tortilla, slice in half if desired, and serve immediately.
8. Enjoy the nutritious and flavorful Salmon and Avocado Wrap with Whole Grain Tortilla.

Nutritional Value (Approx.): Calories: 400 | Protein: 25g | Fiber: 8g | Healthy Fats: 20g | Carbohydrates: 30g

Mediterranean Chickpea Salad

Prep Time: 15 minutes | **Cook Time:** 0 minutes | **Per Serving:** 1 serving

Ingredients:

- 1 can (15 oz) chickpeas, drained and rinsed
- 1 cucumber, diced
- 1 cup cherry tomatoes, halved
- 1/2 red onion, thinly sliced
- 1/2 cup Kalamata olives, pitted and sliced
- 1/4 cup fresh parsley, chopped
- 2 tablespoons extra virgin olive oil
- 1 tablespoon red wine vinegar
- 1 teaspoon dried oregano
- Salt and pepper, to taste
- Crumbled feta cheese (optional)

Instructions:

1. In a large bowl, combine chickpeas, cucumber, cherry tomatoes, red onion, Kalamata olives, and parsley.
2. Drizzle with olive oil and red wine vinegar.
3. Sprinkle with dried oregano, salt, and pepper.
4. Toss gently to combine.
5. If desired, sprinkle with crumbled feta cheese.
6. Serve immediately or refrigerate until ready to serve.
7. Enjoy the refreshing and flavorful Mediterranean Chickpea Salad.

Nutritional Value (Approx. per serving): Calories: 300 | Protein: 10g | Fiber: 10g | Healthy Fats: 12g | Carbohydrates: 40g

Turkey and Vegetable Stir-Fry with Brown Rice

Prep Time: 15 minutes | **Cook Time:** 15 minutes | **Per Serving:** 1 serving

Ingredients:

- 4 oz turkey breast, thinly sliced
- 1 cup mixed vegetables (bell peppers, broccoli, carrots)
- 1 clove garlic, minced
- 1 tablespoon soy sauce (or tamari for gluten-free)
- 1 tablespoon hoisin sauce
- 1 tablespoon olive oil
- Cooked brown rice, for serving
- Sesame seeds and sliced green onions, for garnish

Instructions:

1. Heat olive oil in a large skillet or wok over medium-high heat.
2. Add minced garlic and sauté until fragrant.
3. Add sliced turkey breast and stir-fry until cooked through.
4. Add mixed vegetables and stir-fry for another 3-5 minutes until vegetables are tender-crisp.
5. Stir in soy sauce and hoisin sauce, tossing to coat evenly.
6. Remove from heat.
7. Serve turkey and vegetable stir-fry over cooked brown rice.
8. Garnish with sesame seeds and sliced green onions.
9. Enjoy the savory and satisfying Turkey and Vegetable Stir-Fry with Brown Rice.

Nutritional Value (Approx. per serving): Calories: 400 | Protein: 30g | Fiber: 8g | Healthy Fats: 10g | Carbohydrates: 50g

Sweet Potato and Black Bean Tacos with Cilantro Lime Slaw

Prep Time: 20 minutes | **Cook Time:** 30 minutes | **Per Serving:** Makes 4 tacos

Ingredients:

- 2 medium sweet potatoes, peeled and diced

- 1 can (15 oz) black beans, drained and rinsed

- 1 tablespoon olive oil

- 1 teaspoon chili powder

- 1/2 teaspoon ground cumin

- Salt and pepper, to taste

- 4 small corn or flour tortillas

- For the Cilantro Lime Slaw:

    o 1 cup shredded cabbage or coleslaw mix

    o 2 tablespoons Greek yogurt or mayo

    o Juice of 1 lime

    o 2 tablespoons fresh cilantro, chopped

- Optional toppings: Sliced avocado, salsa, hot sauce

Instructions:

1. Preheat oven to 400°F (200°C).

2. Toss diced sweet potatoes with olive oil, chili powder, cumin, salt, and pepper on a baking sheet.

3. Roast in the oven for 25-30 minutes until tender and lightly browned.

4. In a bowl, combine black beans with a pinch of salt and set aside.

5. In another bowl, mix shredded cabbage or coleslaw mix with Greek yogurt or mayo, lime juice, and chopped cilantro to make the slaw.

6. Heat tortillas in a dry skillet until warmed through.

7. Assemble tacos by filling each tortilla with roasted sweet potatoes, black beans, and cilantro lime slaw.

8. Add optional toppings if desired.

9. Serve immediately and enjoy the delicious Sweet Potato and Black Bean Tacos with Cilantro Lime Slaw.

Nutritional Value (Approx. per taco): Calories: 300 | Protein: 10g | Fiber: 8g | Healthy Fats: 5g | Carbohydrates: 50g

Buddha Bowl with Roasted Vegetables and Tahini Dressing

Prep Time: 20 minutes | **Cook Time:** 30 minutes | **Per Serving:** 1 serving

Ingredients:

- 1 cup cooked quinoa or brown rice
- 1 cup mixed greens (spinach, kale)
- 1/2 cup roasted sweet potatoes, cubed
- 1/2 cup roasted chickpeas
- 1/2 cup cherry tomatoes, halved
- 1/4 cup cucumber, sliced
- 2 tablespoons tahini
- Juice of 1 lemon
- 1 tablespoon olive oil
- Salt and pepper, to taste
- Optional toppings: Avocado slices, sesame seeds, fresh herbs

Instructions:

1. Preheat oven to 400°F (200°C).
2. Toss sweet potatoes with olive oil, salt, and pepper on a baking sheet.
3. Roast in the oven for 20-25 minutes until tender and lightly browned.
4. Toss chickpeas with olive oil, salt, and pepper on another baking sheet.
5. Roast chickpeas in the oven for 15-20 minutes until crispy.
6. In a bowl, whisk together tahini, lemon juice, olive oil, salt, and pepper to make the dressing.
7. Assemble Buddha bowl by layering cooked quinoa or brown rice, mixed greens, roasted sweet potatoes, roasted chickpeas, cherry tomatoes, and cucumber.
8. Drizzle with tahini dressing.
9. Add optional toppings if desired.

10. Serve immediately and enjoy the nourishing Buddha Bowl with Roasted Vegetables and Tahini Dressing.

Nutritional Value (Approx. per serving): Calories: 400 | Protein: 12g | Fiber: 10g | Healthy Fats: 15g | Carbohydrates: 55g

Chapter 6: Dinner Recipes

Roasted Salmon with Asparagus and Lemon

Prep Time: 10 minutes | **Cook Time:** 20 minutes | **Per Serving:** 1 serving

Ingredients:

- 4 oz salmon fillet
- 1 cup asparagus, trimmed
- 1 lemon, sliced
- 1 tablespoon olive oil
- Salt and pepper, to taste
- Fresh dill, chopped (optional)

Instructions:

1. Preheat oven to 400°F (200°C).
2. Place salmon fillet and asparagus on a baking sheet lined with parchment paper.
3. Drizzle with olive oil and season with salt and pepper.
4. Arrange lemon slices on top of salmon and asparagus.
5. Roast in the oven for 15-20 minutes until salmon is cooked through and asparagus is tender.
6. Sprinkle with fresh dill if desired.
7. Serve immediately and enjoy the light and flavorful Roasted Salmon with Asparagus and Lemon.

Nutritional Value (Approx.): Calories: 300 | Protein: 25g | Fiber: 4g | Healthy Fats: 18g | Carbohydrates: 10g

Vegetable Stir-Fry with Tofu

Prep Time: 15 minutes | **Cook Time:** 15 minutes | **Per Serving:** 1 serving

Ingredients:

- 4 oz firm tofu, cubed
- 1 cup mixed vegetables (bell peppers, broccoli, snap peas)
- 1 clove garlic, minced
- 1 tablespoon soy sauce (or tamari for gluten-free)
- 1 tablespoon hoisin sauce
- 1 tablespoon olive oil
- Cooked brown rice, for serving
- Sesame seeds and sliced green onions, for garnish

Instructions:

1. Heat olive oil in a large skillet or wok over medium-high heat.
2. Add minced garlic and sauté until fragrant.
3. Add cubed tofu and stir-fry until golden brown.
4. Add mixed vegetables and stir-fry for another 3-5 minutes until vegetables are tender-crisp.
5. Stir in soy sauce and hoisin sauce, tossing to coat evenly.
6. Remove from heat.
7. Serve vegetable stir-fry with tofu over cooked brown rice.
8. Garnish with sesame seeds and sliced green onions.
9. Enjoy the delicious and nutritious Vegetable Stir-Fry with Tofu.

Nutritional Value (Approx. per serving): Calories: 350 | Protein: 15g | Fiber: 8g | Healthy Fats: 15g | Carbohydrates: 45g

Quinoa and Kale Stuffed Portobello Mushrooms

Prep Time: 15 minutes | **Cook Time:** 20 minutes | **Per Serving:** 1 serving

Ingredients:

- 2 large portobello mushrooms, stems removed
- 1/2 cup quinoa, cooked
- 1 cup kale, chopped
- 1/4 cup cherry tomatoes, diced
- 1/4 cup feta cheese, crumbled (optional)
- 1 tablespoon olive oil
- 1 clove garlic, minced
- Salt and pepper, to taste

Instructions:

1. Preheat oven to 375°F (190°C).
2. Brush portobello mushrooms with olive oil and place on a baking sheet.
3. In a skillet, heat olive oil over medium heat.
4. Add minced garlic and sauté until fragrant.
5. Stir in chopped kale and cook until wilted.
6. Remove from heat and mix in cooked quinoa, cherry tomatoes, and feta cheese if using.
7. Season with salt and pepper.
8. Spoon quinoa mixture into portobello mushrooms.
9. Bake for 15-20 minutes until mushrooms are tender.
10. Serve warm and enjoy the hearty Quinoa and Kale Stuffed Portobello Mushrooms.

Nutritional Value (Approx. per serving): Calories: 350 | Protein: 15g | Fiber: 10g | Healthy Fats: 12g | Carbohydrates: 45g

Grilled Chicken with Quinoa Salad

Prep Time: 15 minutes | **Cook Time:** 15 minutes | **Per Serving:** 1 serving

Ingredients:

- 4 oz chicken breast, grilled and sliced
- 1/2 cup quinoa, cooked
- 1/2 cup cucumber, diced
- 1/2 cup cherry tomatoes, halved
- 1/4 cup red onion, thinly sliced
- 1/4 cup fresh parsley, chopped
- 2 tablespoons olive oil
- 1 tablespoon lemon juice
- Salt and pepper, to taste

Instructions:

1. Season chicken breast with salt and pepper, then grill until fully cooked. Slice thinly.
2. In a large bowl, combine cooked quinoa, cucumber, cherry tomatoes, red onion, and parsley.
3. Drizzle with olive oil and lemon juice.
4. Season with salt and pepper.
5. Toss gently to combine.
6. Top quinoa salad with grilled chicken slices.
7. Serve immediately and enjoy the fresh and nutritious Grilled Chicken with Quinoa Salad.

Nutritional Value (Approx. per serving): Calories: 400 | Protein: 30g | Fiber: 8g | Healthy Fats: 15g | Carbohydrates: 35g

Chickpea and Spinach Curry

Prep Time: 10 minutes | **Cook Time:** 20 minutes | **Per Serving:** 1 serving

Ingredients:

- 1 can (15 oz) chickpeas, drained and rinsed
- 2 cups fresh spinach
- 1 onion, chopped
- 2 cloves garlic, minced
- 1 tablespoon ginger, minced
- 1 can (14 oz) diced tomatoes
- 1 cup coconut milk
- 1 tablespoon curry powder
- 1 teaspoon ground cumin
- 1 teaspoon turmeric
- 1 tablespoon olive oil
- Salt and pepper, to taste
- Cooked brown rice, for serving

Instructions:

1. Heat olive oil in a large pot over medium heat.
2. Add chopped onion and sauté until softened.
3. Stir in minced garlic and ginger, cooking for 1 minute until fragrant.
4. Add curry powder, cumin, and turmeric, stirring to combine.
5. Pour in diced tomatoes and coconut milk, bringing to a simmer.
6. Add chickpeas and simmer for 10 minutes.
7. Stir in fresh spinach and cook until wilted.
8. Season with salt and pepper to taste.
9. Serve curry over cooked brown rice.
10. Enjoy the rich and flavorful Chickpea and Spinach Curry.

Nutritional Value (Approx. per serving): Calories: 350 | Protein: 12g | Fiber: 10g | Healthy Fats: 15g | Carbohydrates: 45g

Turkey Meatballs with Zucchini Noodles

Prep Time: 15 minutes | **Cook Time:** 20 minutes | **Per Serving:** 1 serving

Ingredients:

- 4 oz ground turkey
- 1/4 cup breadcrumbs (optional)
- 1 egg
- 2 cloves garlic, minced
- 1 tablespoon fresh parsley, chopped
- 1 tablespoon olive oil
- Salt and pepper, to taste
- 2 medium zucchinis, spiralized
- Marinara sauce, for serving

Instructions:

1. In a bowl, combine ground turkey, breadcrumbs (if using), egg, minced garlic, parsley, salt, and pepper.
2. Mix until well combined and form into small meatballs.
3. Heat olive oil in a skillet over medium heat.
4. Cook meatballs until browned on all sides and cooked through, about 10-15 minutes.
5. In another skillet, lightly sauté zucchini noodles until tender.
6. Serve turkey meatballs over zucchini noodles with marinara sauce.
7. Enjoy the light and satisfying Turkey Meatballs with Zucchini Noodles.

Nutritional Value (Approx. per serving): Calories: 350 | Protein: 25g | Fiber: 6g | Healthy Fats: 15g | Carbohydrates: 20g

Baked Cod with Garlic and Herbs

Prep Time: 10 minutes | **Cook Time:** 15 minutes | **Per Serving:** 1 serving

Ingredients:

- 4 oz cod fillet
- 2 cloves garlic, minced
- 1 tablespoon fresh parsley, chopped
- 1 tablespoon fresh lemon juice
- 1 tablespoon olive oil
- Salt and pepper, to taste
- Lemon wedges, for serving

Instructions:

1. Preheat oven to 400°F (200°C).
2. Place cod fillet on a baking sheet lined with parchment paper.
3. In a small bowl, mix minced garlic, parsley, lemon juice, olive oil, salt, and pepper.
4. Spread the garlic and herb mixture over the cod fillet.
5. Bake in the oven for 12-15 minutes until the fish is cooked through and flakes easily with a fork.
6. Serve with lemon wedges.
7. Enjoy the delicate and flavorful Baked Cod with Garlic and Herbs.

Nutritional Value (Approx. per serving): Calories: 200 | Protein: 25g | Fiber: 1g | Healthy Fats: 10g | Carbohydrates: 5g

Vegetarian Chili with Beans and Sweet Potatoes

Prep Time: 15 minutes | **Cook Time:** 40 minutes | **Per Serving:** 1 serving

Ingredients:

- 1 can (15 oz) black beans, drained and rinsed
- 1 can (15 oz) kidney beans, drained and rinsed
- 1 large sweet potato, peeled and diced
- 1 onion, chopped
- 2 cloves garlic, minced
- 1 can (14 oz) diced tomatoes
- 1 cup vegetable broth
- 1 tablespoon chili powder
- 1 teaspoon ground cumin
- 1 teaspoon smoked paprika
- 1 tablespoon olive oil
- Salt and pepper, to taste

Instructions:

1. Heat olive oil in a large pot over medium heat.
2. Add chopped onion and sauté until softened.
3. Stir in minced garlic, chili powder, cumin, and smoked paprika, cooking for 1 minute until fragrant.
4. Add diced sweet potato, black beans, kidney beans, diced tomatoes, and vegetable broth.
5. Bring to a boil, then reduce heat to low and simmer for 30-35 minutes until sweet potatoes are tender.
6. Season with salt and pepper to taste.
7. Serve hot and enjoy the hearty and nutritious Vegetarian Chili with Beans and Sweet Potatoes.

Nutritional Value (Approx. per serving): Calories: 400 | Protein: 15g | Fiber: 15g | Healthy Fats: 8g | Carbohydrates: 70g

Chapter 7: Snack Recipes

Greek Yogurt with Honey and Walnuts

Prep Time: 5 minutes | **Cook Time:** 0 minutes | **Per Serving:** 1 serving

Ingredients:

- 1 cup Greek yogurt
- 1 tablespoon honey
- 2 tablespoons chopped walnuts

Instructions:

1. Scoop Greek yogurt into a bowl.
2. Drizzle honey over the yogurt.
3. Sprinkle chopped walnuts on top.
4. Serve immediately and enjoy.

Nutritional Value (Approx.): Calories: 250 | Protein: 15g | Fiber: 2g | Healthy Fats: 10g | Carbohydrates: 20g

Dark Chocolate Squares

Prep Time: 0 minutes | **Cook Time:** 0 minutes | **Per Serving:** 1 serving

Ingredients:

- 1 oz dark chocolate (70% cocoa or higher)

Instructions:

1. Break dark chocolate into squares.
2. Serve immediately and enjoy.

Nutritional Value (Approx.): Calories: 150 | Protein: 2g | Fiber: 3g | Healthy Fats: 12g | Carbohydrates: 10g

Carrot and Hummus Sticks

Prep Time: 10 minutes | **Cook Time:** 0 minutes | **Per Serving:** 1 serving

Ingredients:

- 2 medium carrots, peeled and cut into sticks
- 1/4 cup hummus

Instructions:

1. Peel and cut carrots into sticks.
2. Place carrot sticks on a plate.
3. Serve with a side of hummus for dipping.
4. Enjoy this crunchy and nutritious snack.

Nutritional Value (Approx.): Calories: 150 | Protein: 4g | Fiber: 6g | Healthy Fats: 6g | Carbohydrates: 18g

Apple Slices with Almond Butter

Prep Time: 5 minutes | **Cook Time:** 0 minutes | **Per Serving:** 1 serving

Ingredients:

- 1 medium apple, cored and sliced
- 2 tablespoons almond butter

Instructions:

1. Core and slice the apple.
2. Spread almond butter on each apple slice.
3. Serve immediately and enjoy.

Nutritional Value (Approx.): Calories: 200 | Protein: 4g | Fiber: 5g | Healthy Fats: 12g | Carbohydrates: 24g

Mixed Nuts and Seeds

Prep Time: 0 minutes | **Cook Time:** 0 minutes | **Per Serving:** 1 serving

Ingredients:

- 1/4 cup mixed nuts (almonds, walnuts, cashews)
- 1/4 cup mixed seeds (pumpkin seeds, sunflower seeds, chia seeds)

Instructions:

1. Combine mixed nuts and seeds in a small bowl.
2. Serve immediately and enjoy.

Nutritional Value (Approx.): Calories: 200 | Protein: 7g | Fiber: 4g | Healthy Fats: 16g | Carbohydrates: 8g

Fresh Fruit Salad

Prep Time: 10 minutes | **Cook Time:** 0 minutes | **Per Serving:** 1 serving

Ingredients:

- 1/2 cup strawberries, sliced
- 1/2 cup blueberries
- 1/2 cup pineapple, diced
- 1/2 cup kiwi, diced

Instructions:

1. Wash and prepare the fruits.
2. Combine all the fruits in a bowl.
3. Mix gently and serve immediately.

Nutritional Value (Approx.): Calories: 100 | Protein: 2g | Fiber: 4g | Healthy Fats: 0g | Carbohydrates: 25g

Celery Sticks with Peanut Butter

Prep Time: 5 minutes | **Cook Time:** 0 minutes | **Per Serving:** 1 serving

Ingredients:

- 3 celery stalks, cut into sticks
- 2 tablespoons peanut butter

Instructions:

1. Cut celery stalks into sticks.
2. Spread peanut butter on each celery stick.
3. Serve immediately and enjoy.

Nutritional Value (Approx.): Calories: 180 | Protein: 6g | Fiber: 4g | Healthy Fats: 14g | Carbohydrates: 10g

Kale Chips

Prep Time: 10 minutes | **Cook Time:** 15 minutes | **Per Serving:** 1 serving

Ingredients:

- 2 cups kale leaves, washed and dried
- 1 tablespoon olive oil
- 1/4 teaspoon sea salt

Instructions:

1. Preheat oven to 350°F (175°C).
2. Tear kale leaves into bite-sized pieces.
3. Toss kale with olive oil and sea salt.
4. Spread kale on a baking sheet in a single layer.
5. Bake for 10-15 minutes until crispy.
6. Allow to cool slightly and serve.

Nutritional Value (Approx.): Calories: 80 | Protein: 2g | Fiber: 2g | Healthy Fats: 7g | Carbohydrates: 3g

Chapter 8: Smoothie Recipes

Green Revitalizer Smoothie

Prep Time: 5 minutes | **Cook Time:** 0 minutes | **Per Serving:** 1 serving

Ingredients:

- 1 cup spinach leaves (fresh or frozen)
- 1/2 cucumber, peeled and sliced
- 1/2 green apple, cored and chopped
- 1/2 lemon, juiced
- 1 tablespoon chia seeds
- 1 cup unsweetened almond milk
- Ice cubes (optional)

Instructions:

1. Combine spinach, cucumber, green apple, lemon juice, chia seeds, and almond milk in a blender.
2. Blend until smooth and creamy.
3. Add ice cubes if desired and blend again.
4. Pour into a glass and enjoy the refreshing Green Revitalizer Smoothie.

Nutritional Value (Approx.): Calories: 200 | Protein: 6g | Fiber: 4g | Healthy Fats: 8g | Carbohydrates: 25g

Berry Banana Smoothie

Prep Time: 5 minutes | **Cook Time:** 0 minutes | **Per Serving:** 1 serving

Ingredients:

- 1/2 cup strawberries

- 1/2 cup blueberries

- 1/2 banana

- 1/2 cup Greek yogurt

- 1/2 cup unsweetened almond milk

- 1 tablespoon flaxseeds

Instructions:

1. Combine strawberries, blueberries, banana, Greek yogurt, almond milk, and flaxseeds in a blender.

2. Blend until smooth and creamy.

3. Pour into a glass and enjoy this antioxidant-rich smoothie.

Nutritional Value (Approx.): Calories: 250 | Protein: 10g | Fiber: 5g | Healthy Fats: 7g | Carbohydrates: 40g

Tropical Mango Smoothie

Prep Time: 5 minutes | **Cook Time:** 0 minutes | **Per Serving:** 1 serving

Ingredients:

- 1 cup mango chunks (fresh or frozen)
- 1/2 cup pineapple chunks (fresh or frozen)
- 1/2 banana
- 1/2 cup coconut water
- 1 tablespoon hemp seeds

Instructions:

1. Combine mango, pineapple, banana, coconut water, and hemp seeds in a blender.
2. Blend until smooth and creamy.
3. Pour into a glass and enjoy this tropical treat.

Nutritional Value (Approx.): Calories: 210 | Protein: 4g | Fiber: 4g | Healthy Fats: 5g | Carbohydrates: 45g

Peanut Butter Banana Smoothie

Prep Time: 5 minutes | **Cook Time:** 0 minutes | **Per Serving:** 1 serving

Ingredients:

- 1 banana
- 1 tablespoon peanut butter
- 1/2 cup Greek yogurt
- 1/2 cup unsweetened almond milk
- 1 tablespoon honey
- Ice cubes (optional)

Instructions:

1. Combine banana, peanut butter, Greek yogurt, almond milk, and honey in a blender.
2. Blend until smooth and creamy.
3. Add ice cubes if desired and blend again.
4. Pour into a glass and enjoy this protein-packed smoothie.

Nutritional Value (Approx.): Calories: 300 | Protein: 12g | Fiber: 3g | Healthy Fats: 12g | Carbohydrates: 40g

Avocado Spinach Smoothie

Prep Time: 5 minutes | **Cook Time:** 0 minutes | **Per Serving:** 1 serving

Ingredients:

- 1/2 avocado
- 1 cup spinach leaves (fresh or frozen)
- 1/2 banana
- 1/2 cup coconut milk
- 1 tablespoon chia seeds
- Ice cubes (optional)

Instructions:

1. Combine avocado, spinach, banana, coconut milk, and chia seeds in a blender.
2. Blend until smooth and creamy.
3. Add ice cubes if desired and blend again.
4. Pour into a glass and enjoy this creamy and nutritious smoothie.

Nutritional Value (Approx.): Calories: 250 | Protein: 4g | Fiber: 8g | Healthy Fats: 18g | Carbohydrates: 22g

Chocolate Almond Smoothie

Prep Time: 5 minutes | **Cook Time:** 0 minutes | **Per Serving:** 1 serving

Ingredients:

- 1 banana
- 1 tablespoon almond butter
- 1 tablespoon unsweetened cocoa powder
- 1/2 cup unsweetened almond milk
- 1/2 cup Greek yogurt
- Ice cubes (optional)

Instructions:

1. Combine banana, almond butter, cocoa powder, almond milk, and Greek yogurt in a blender.
2. Blend until smooth and creamy.
3. Add ice cubes if desired and blend again.
4. Pour into a glass and enjoy this delicious chocolate treat.

Nutritional Value (Approx.): Calories: 300 | Protein: 12g | Fiber: 5g | Healthy Fats: 14g | Carbohydrates: 35g

Berry Green Smoothie

Prep Time: 5 minutes | **Cook Time:** 0 minutes | **Per Serving:** 1 serving

Ingredients:

- 1/2 cup blueberries
- 1/2 cup raspberries
- 1 cup spinach leaves (fresh or frozen)
- 1/2 cup Greek yogurt
- 1/2 cup unsweetened almond milk
- 1 tablespoon flaxseeds

Instructions:

1. Combine blueberries, raspberries, spinach, Greek yogurt, almond milk, and flaxseeds in a blender.

2. Blend until smooth and creamy.

3. Pour into a glass and enjoy this berry-packed green smoothie.

Nutritional Value (Approx.): Calories: 250 | Protein: 10g | Fiber: 6g | Healthy Fats: 7g | Carbohydrates: 40g

Citrus Ginger Smoothie

Prep Time: 5 minutes | **Cook Time:** 0 minutes | **Per Serving:** 1 serving

Ingredients:

- 1 orange, peeled and segmented
- 1/2 lemon, juiced
- 1 small piece of ginger, peeled and grated
- 1/2 banana
- 1/2 cup Greek yogurt
- 1/2 cup coconut water
- Ice cubes (optional)

Instructions:

1. Combine orange, lemon juice, ginger, banana, Greek yogurt, and coconut water in a blender.
2. Blend until smooth and creamy.
3. Add ice cubes if desired and blend again.
4. Pour into a glass and enjoy this zesty and refreshing smoothie.

Nutritional Value (Approx.): Calories: 200 | Protein: 8g | Fiber: 3g | Healthy Fats: 4g | Carbohydrates: 35g

Chapter 9: Dessert Recipes

Chia Seed Pudding with Berries

Prep Time: 10 minutes | **Cook Time:** 0 minutes | **Per Serving:** 4 servings

Ingredients:

- 1 cup almond milk
- 1/4 cup chia seeds
- 1 tablespoon maple syrup
- 1/2 teaspoon vanilla extract
- 1 cup mixed berries (strawberries, blueberries, raspberries)

Instructions:

1. In a bowl, combine almond milk, chia seeds, maple syrup, and vanilla extract.
2. Stir well to combine.
3. Cover and refrigerate for at least 4 hours or overnight.
4. Before serving, give it a good stir and top with mixed berries.
5. Serve chilled and enjoy.

Nutritional Value (Approx.): Calories: 150 | Protein: 4g | Fiber: 8g | Healthy Fats: 8g | Carbohydrates: 18g

Avocado Chocolate Mousse

Prep Time: 10 minutes | **Cook Time:** 0 minutes | **Per Serving:** 4 servings

Ingredients:

- 2 ripe avocados
- 1/4 cup unsweetened cocoa powder
- 1/4 cup maple syrup
- 1/4 cup almond milk
- 1 teaspoon vanilla extract
- Pinch of sea salt

Instructions:

1. Scoop the flesh of the avocados into a blender.
2. Add cocoa powder, maple syrup, almond milk, vanilla extract, and sea salt.
3. Blend until smooth and creamy.
4. Spoon into serving dishes and refrigerate for at least 30 minutes before serving.
5. Serve chilled and enjoy this decadent mousse.

Nutritional Value (Approx.): Calories: 200 | Protein: 3g | Fiber: 7g | Healthy Fats: 15g | Carbohydrates: 20g

Coconut Macaroons

Prep Time: 10 minutes | **Cook Time:** 20 minutes | **Per Serving:** 12 servings

Ingredients:

- 2 1/2 cups shredded coconut
- 1/2 cup almond flour
- 1/3 cup maple syrup
- 1/4 cup coconut oil, melted
- 1 teaspoon vanilla extract
- Pinch of sea salt

Instructions:

1. Preheat the oven to 325°F (165°C) and line a baking sheet with parchment paper.
2. In a bowl, mix together shredded coconut, almond flour, maple syrup, coconut oil, vanilla extract, and sea salt.
3. Scoop tablespoon-sized mounds onto the prepared baking sheet.
4. Bake for 18-20 minutes, or until golden brown.
5. Allow to cool completely before serving.

Nutritional Value (Approx.): Calories: 150 | Protein: 2g | Fiber: 3g | Healthy Fats: 12g | Carbohydrates: 10g

Berry Parfait

Prep Time: 10 minutes | **Cook Time:** 0 minutes | **Per Serving:** 2 servings

Ingredients:

- 1 cup Greek yogurt
- 1/2 cup granola
- 1 cup mixed berries (strawberries, blueberries, raspberries)
- 1 tablespoon honey

Instructions:

1. In serving glasses, layer Greek yogurt, granola, and mixed berries.
2. Drizzle honey on top.
3. Serve immediately and enjoy this delicious parfait.

Nutritional Value (Approx.): Calories: 300 | Protein: 12g | Fiber: 5g | Healthy Fats: 10g | Carbohydrates: 40g

Baked Apples with Cinnamon

Prep Time: 10 minutes | **Cook Time:** 30 minutes | **Per Serving:** 4 servings

Ingredients:

- 4 medium apples, cored
- 1/4 cup raisins
- 1/4 cup chopped walnuts
- 1 tablespoon cinnamon
- 1 tablespoon maple syrup
- 1/2 cup water

Instructions:

1. Preheat the oven to 350°F (175°C).
2. In a bowl, mix raisins, walnuts, cinnamon, and maple syrup.
3. Stuff the mixture into the cored apples.
4. Place apples in a baking dish and add water to the bottom.
5. Bake for 30 minutes or until apples are tender.
6. Serve warm and enjoy.

Nutritional Value (Approx.): Calories: 200 | Protein: 2g | Fiber: 6g | Healthy Fats: 7g | Carbohydrates: 35g

Dark Chocolate Bark with Nuts and Seeds

Prep Time: 10 minutes | **Cook Time:** 5 minutes | **Per Serving:** 8 servings

Ingredients:

- 8 oz dark chocolate (70% cocoa or higher)
- 1/4 cup almonds, chopped
- 1/4 cup pumpkin seeds
- 1/4 cup dried cranberries
- 1 tablespoon chia seeds

Instructions:

1. Melt dark chocolate in a double boiler or microwave.
2. Spread melted chocolate evenly on a parchment-lined baking sheet.
3. Sprinkle with almonds, pumpkin seeds, dried cranberries, and chia seeds.
4. Refrigerate until set, about 30 minutes.
5. Break into pieces and serve.

Nutritional Value (Approx.): Calories: 200 | Protein: 3g | Fiber: 4g | Healthy Fats: 14g | Carbohydrates: 20g

Mango Sorbet

Prep Time: 10 minutes | **Cook Time:** 0 minutes | **Per Serving:** 4 servings

Ingredients:

- 3 cups frozen mango chunks
- 1/4 cup coconut milk
- 1 tablespoon lime juice
- 1 tablespoon honey

Instructions:

1. Combine frozen mango, coconut milk, lime juice, and honey in a blender.
2. Blend until smooth and creamy.
3. Serve immediately or freeze for a firmer texture.
4. Enjoy this refreshing sorbet.

Nutritional Value (Approx.): Calories: 120 | Protein: 1g | Fiber: 3g | Healthy Fats: 2g | Carbohydrates: 26g

Almond Flour Brownies

Prep Time: 15 minutes | **Cook Time:** 25 minutes | **Per Serving:** 12 servings

Ingredients:

- 1 cup almond flour
- 1/4 cup cocoa powder
- 1/2 cup coconut sugar
- 1/4 cup coconut oil, melted
- 2 large eggs
- 1 teaspoon vanilla extract
- 1/2 teaspoon baking soda
- 1/4 teaspoon sea salt

Instructions:

1. Preheat the oven to 350°F (175°C) and line an 8x8-inch baking pan with parchment paper.
2. In a bowl, mix almond flour, cocoa powder, coconut sugar, baking soda, and sea salt.
3. In another bowl, whisk together melted coconut oil, eggs, and vanilla extract.
4. Combine the wet and dry ingredients and mix until smooth.
5. Pour batter into the prepared pan and spread evenly.
6. Bake for 20-25 minutes or until a toothpick inserted comes out clean.
7. Allow to cool before cutting into squares.

Nutritional Value (Approx.): Calories: 160 | Protein: 4g | Fiber: 3g | Healthy Fats: 12g | Carbohydrates: 12g

Chapter 10: Regional and Global Specialties

American Recipes

Classic Cobb Salad

Prep Time: 20 minutes | **Cook Time:** 0 minutes | **Per Serving:** 1 serving

Ingredients:

- 2 cups mixed greens (romaine, iceberg, watercress)
- 1/2 avocado, diced
- 2 hard-boiled eggs, chopped
- 4 oz cooked chicken breast, diced
- 2 slices cooked bacon, crumbled
- 1/2 cup cherry tomatoes, halved
- 1/4 cup blue cheese, crumbled
- 1/4 cup red onion, thinly sliced
- 2 tablespoons olive oil
- 1 tablespoon red wine vinegar
- Salt and pepper, to taste

Instructions:

1. Arrange mixed greens on a large plate or in a salad bowl.
2. Top with diced avocado, chopped hard-boiled eggs, diced chicken breast, crumbled bacon, cherry tomatoes, blue cheese, and red onion.
3. Drizzle olive oil and red wine vinegar over the salad.
4. Season with salt and pepper to taste.
5. Toss gently to combine.
6. Serve immediately and enjoy the classic flavors of the Cobb Salad.

Nutritional Value (Approx. per serving): Calories: 450 | Protein: 30g | Fiber: 10g | Healthy Fats: 30g | Carbohydrates: 10g

Barbecue Pulled Pork Sandwiches

Prep Time: 15 minutes | **Cook Time:** 6 hours (slow cooker) | **Per Serving:** 1 serving

Ingredients:

- 4 oz pork shoulder
- 1/2 cup barbecue sauce
- 1 whole wheat hamburger bun
- 1/4 cup coleslaw (optional)
- 1 tablespoon olive oil
- Salt and pepper, to taste

Instructions:

1. Season pork shoulder with salt and pepper.
2. Heat olive oil in a skillet over medium-high heat.
3. Sear pork shoulder on all sides until browned.
4. Transfer pork to a slow cooker and pour barbecue sauce over it.
5. Cook on low for 6 hours or until pork is tender and easily shredded.
6. Shred pork with two forks and mix with remaining barbecue sauce in the slow cooker.
7. Serve pulled pork on a whole wheat hamburger bun with coleslaw, if desired.
8. Enjoy the savory and tender Barbecue Pulled Pork Sandwich.

Nutritional Value (Approx. per serving): Calories: 450 | Protein: 25g | Fiber: 3g | Healthy Fats: 18g | Carbohydrates: 40g

New England Clam Chowder

Prep Time: 15 minutes | **Cook Time:** 30 minutes | **Per Serving:** 1 serving

Ingredients:

- 4 oz clams, chopped (canned or fresh)
- 1 cup potatoes, diced
- 1/2 cup onion, chopped
- 1/2 cup celery, chopped
- 1/4 cup carrots, diced
- 1 cup clam juice
- 1 cup milk
- 1 tablespoon butter
- 1 tablespoon flour
- 1 bay leaf
- Salt and pepper, to taste

Instructions:

1. In a large pot, melt butter over medium heat.
2. Add chopped onion, celery, and carrots. Sauté until softened.
3. Stir in flour and cook for 1-2 minutes.
4. Add diced potatoes, clam juice, and bay leaf. Bring to a boil.
5. Reduce heat and simmer for 15-20 minutes until potatoes are tender.
6. Add chopped clams and milk. Heat through but do not boil.
7. Season with salt and pepper to taste.
8. Remove bay leaf before serving.
9. Serve hot and enjoy the creamy and comforting New England Clam Chowder.

Nutritional Value (Approx. per serving): Calories: 300 | Protein: 15g | Fiber: 3g | Healthy Fats: 12g | Carbohydrates: 35g

Southern Shrimp and Grits

Prep Time: 15 minutes | **Cook Time:** 30 minutes | **Per Serving:** 1 serving

Ingredients:

- 4 oz shrimp, peeled and deveined
- 1/2 cup grits
- 2 cups water
- 1/2 cup cheddar cheese, shredded
- 2 slices bacon, chopped
- 1/4 cup green onions, chopped
- 1 tablespoon butter
- 1 tablespoon olive oil
- 1 clove garlic, minced
- Salt and pepper, to taste

Instructions:

1. In a pot, bring water to a boil. Add grits and reduce heat to low.
2. Cook grits, stirring frequently, until thickened, about 20-25 minutes.
3. Stir in butter and shredded cheddar cheese. Season with salt and pepper. Set aside.
4. In a skillet, cook chopped bacon over medium heat until crispy. Remove bacon and set aside.
5. In the same skillet, add olive oil and minced garlic. Sauté until fragrant.
6. Add shrimp and cook until pink and opaque, about 3-4 minutes.
7. Stir in cooked bacon and chopped green onions.
8. Serve shrimp mixture over the cheesy grits.
9. Enjoy the rich and flavorful Southern Shrimp and Grits.

Nutritional Value (Approx. per serving): Calories: 450 | Protein: 25g | Fiber: 2g | Healthy Fats: 25g | Carbohydrates: 35g

California Turkey Avocado Wrap

Prep Time: 10 minutes | **Cook Time:** 0 minutes | **Per Serving:** 1 serving

Ingredients:

- 1 whole wheat tortilla
- 4 oz turkey breast, sliced
- 1/2 avocado, sliced
- 1/2 cup mixed greens
- 1/4 cup cherry tomatoes, halved
- 1 tablespoon hummus
- Salt and pepper, to taste

Instructions:

1. Lay the whole wheat tortilla on a flat surface.
2. Spread hummus evenly over the tortilla.
3. Layer sliced turkey breast, avocado, mixed greens, and cherry tomatoes.
4. Season with salt and pepper to taste.
5. Roll the tortilla tightly to form a wrap.
6. Slice in half if desired and serve immediately.
7. Enjoy the fresh and delicious California Turkey Avocado Wrap.

Nutritional Value (Approx. per serving): Calories: 350 | Protein: 25g | Fiber: 10g | Healthy Fats: 15g | Carbohydrates: 35g

Tex-Mex Chicken Enchiladas

Prep Time: 20 minutes | **Cook Time:** 30 minutes | **Per Serving:** 1 serving

Ingredients:

- 4 oz cooked chicken breast, shredded
- 1/2 cup enchilada sauce
- 1/2 cup black beans, drained and rinsed
- 1/4 cup corn kernels
- 1/4 cup cheddar cheese, shredded
- 2 corn tortillas
- 1/4 cup green onions, chopped
- 1 tablespoon olive oil
- Salt and pepper, to taste

Instructions:

1. Preheat oven to 350°F (175°C).
2. In a bowl, mix shredded chicken, black beans, corn, and 1/4 cup enchilada sauce. Season with salt and pepper.
3. Heat corn tortillas in a skillet until pliable.
4. Fill each tortilla with the chicken mixture and roll up.
5. Place enchiladas in a baking dish and pour remaining enchilada sauce over the top.
6. Sprinkle with shredded cheddar cheese.
7. Bake for 20-25 minutes until cheese is melted and bubbly.
8. Garnish with chopped green onions.
9. Serve hot and enjoy the flavorful Tex-Mex Chicken Enchiladas.

Nutritional Value (Approx. per serving): Calories: 400 | Protein: 30g | Fiber: 10g | Healthy Fats: 15g | Carbohydrates: 35g

Midwest Beef Pot Roast

Prep Time: 15 minutes | **Cook Time:** 3 hours | **Per Serving:** 1 serving

Ingredients:

- 4 oz beef chuck roast
- 1 cup carrots, chopped
- 1 cup potatoes, chopped
- 1/2 cup onion, chopped
- 1 cup beef broth
- 1 tablespoon olive oil
- 1 tablespoon tomato paste
- 1 teaspoon dried thyme
- 1 bay leaf
- Salt and pepper, to taste

Instructions:

1. Preheat oven to 325°F (160°C).
2. Season beef chuck roast with salt and pepper.
3. Heat olive oil in a Dutch oven over medium-high heat.
4. Sear the beef on all sides until browned.
5. Remove beef and set aside.
6. Add chopped onions, carrots, and potatoes to the pot and sauté until slightly softened.
7. Stir in tomato paste and cook for 1-2 minutes.
8. Return beef to the pot and add beef broth, dried thyme, and bay leaf.
9. Cover and transfer to the preheated oven.
10. Cook for 2.5 to 3 hours until the beef is tender and falls apart easily.
11. Remove bay leaf before serving.
12. Serve hot and enjoy the hearty and comforting Midwest Beef Pot Roast.

Nutritional Value (Approx. per serving): Calories: 450 | Protein: 30g | Fiber: 5g | Healthy Fats: 20g | Carbohydrates: 35g

Buttermilk Fried Chicken

Prep Time: 20 minutes | **Cook Time:** 20 minutes | **Per Serving:** 1 serving

Ingredients:

- 1 chicken thigh
- 1 cup buttermilk
- 1 cup all-purpose flour
- 1 teaspoon paprika
- 1 teaspoon garlic powder
- 1 teaspoon salt
- 1/2 teaspoon black pepper
- Vegetable oil, for frying

Instructions:

1. Marinate the chicken thigh in buttermilk for at least 1 hour or overnight.
2. In a bowl, combine flour, paprika, garlic powder, salt, and black pepper.
3. Remove chicken from buttermilk and dredge in the flour mixture until well coated.
4. Heat vegetable oil in a deep skillet over medium-high heat.
5. Fry the chicken until golden brown and cooked through, about 10-12 minutes per side.
6. Remove and drain on paper towels.
7. Serve hot and enjoy the crispy and flavorful Buttermilk Fried Chicken.

Nutritional Value (Approx. per serving): Calories: 500 | Protein: 25g | Fiber: 2g | Healthy Fats: 25g | Carbohydrates: 40g

Italian Caprese Salad

Prep Time: 10 minutes | **Cook Time:** 0 minutes | **Per Serving:** 1 serving

Ingredients:

- 2 large ripe tomatoes, sliced
- 4 oz fresh mozzarella, sliced
- 1/4 cup fresh basil leaves
- 2 tablespoons extra virgin olive oil
- 1 tablespoon balsamic vinegar
- Salt and pepper, to taste

Instructions:

1. Arrange tomato and mozzarella slices alternately on a serving platter.
2. Tuck fresh basil leaves between the slices.
3. Drizzle with extra virgin olive oil and balsamic vinegar.
4. Season with salt and pepper to taste.
5. Serve immediately and enjoy the fresh and classic flavors of Italian Caprese Salad.

Nutritional Value (Approx. per serving): Calories: 300 | Protein: 15g | Fiber: 3g | Healthy Fats: 20g | Carbohydrates: 10g

French Coq au Vin

Prep Time: 20 minutes | **Cook Time:** 2 hours | **Per Serving:** 1 serving

Ingredients:

- 1 chicken thigh
- 1/2 cup red wine
- 1/2 cup chicken broth
- 1/4 cup pearl onions
- 1/4 cup mushrooms, sliced
- 1 slice bacon, chopped
- 1 clove garlic, minced
- 1 tablespoon tomato paste
- 1 teaspoon fresh thyme
- 1 bay leaf
- 1 tablespoon olive oil
- Salt and pepper, to taste

Instructions:

1. Season chicken thigh with salt and pepper.
2. Heat olive oil in a Dutch oven over medium-high heat.
3. Add bacon and cook until crispy. Remove and set aside.
4. Sear chicken thigh in the same pot until browned on both sides. Remove and set aside.
5. Add pearl onions, mushrooms, and minced garlic. Sauté until softened.
6. Stir in tomato paste and cook for 1 minute.
7. Pour in red wine and chicken broth. Add fresh thyme and bay leaf.
8. Return chicken and bacon to the pot.
9. Cover and simmer on low heat for 1.5 to 2 hours until chicken is tender.
10. Remove bay leaf before serving.

11. Serve hot and enjoy the rich and savory French Coq au Vin.

Nutritional Value (Approx. per serving): Calories: 450 | Protein: 25g | Fiber: 2g | Healthy Fats: 25g | Carbohydrates: 15g

Spanish Paella

Prep Time: 20 minutes | **Cook Time:** 40 minutes | **Per Serving:** 1 serving

Ingredients:

- 1/4 cup arborio rice
- 4 oz shrimp, peeled and deveined
- 2 oz chicken breast, diced
- 2 oz chorizo sausage, sliced
- 1/4 cup peas
- 1/4 cup diced tomatoes
- 1/4 cup bell peppers, sliced
- 1/2 onion, chopped
- 1 clove garlic, minced
- 1 cup chicken broth
- 1/2 teaspoon smoked paprika
- 1/4 teaspoon saffron threads
- 1 tablespoon olive oil
- Salt and pepper, to taste

Instructions:

1. Heat olive oil in a large skillet or paella pan over medium heat.
2. Sauté diced chicken breast and chorizo until browned. Remove and set aside.
3. Add chopped onion, bell peppers, and minced garlic. Sauté until softened.
4. Stir in diced tomatoes, smoked paprika, and saffron threads.
5. Add arborio rice and cook, stirring, for 1-2 minutes.

6. Pour in chicken broth and bring to a simmer.

7. Return chicken and chorizo to the pan. Add peas.

8. Arrange shrimp on top of the rice mixture.

9. Cover and cook on low heat for 20-25 minutes until rice is tender and liquid is absorbed.

10. Season with salt and pepper to taste.

11. Serve hot and enjoy the vibrant and flavorful Spanish Paella.

Nutritional Value (Approx. per serving): Calories: 500 | Protein: 30g | Fiber: 5g | Healthy Fats: 20g | Carbohydrates: 45g

Greek Moussaka

Prep Time: 30 minutes | **Cook Time:** 1 hour | **Per Serving:** 1 serving

Ingredients:

- 1/2 eggplant, sliced
- 4 oz ground beef or lamb
- 1/4 cup onion, chopped
- 1/2 cup diced tomatoes
- 1/4 cup tomato sauce
- 1 clove garlic, minced
- 1/4 teaspoon ground cinnamon
- 1/4 teaspoon ground nutmeg
- 1 tablespoon olive oil
- 1 tablespoon butter
- 1 tablespoon flour
- 1/2 cup milk
- 1/4 cup Parmesan cheese, grated
- Salt and pepper, to taste

Instructions:

1. Preheat oven to 350°F (175°C).

2. Sprinkle eggplant slices with salt and let sit for 10 minutes. Rinse and pat dry.

3. Heat olive oil in a skillet over medium heat. Sauté eggplant slices until softened. Set aside.

4. In the same skillet, cook ground beef or lamb until browned. Add chopped onion and minced garlic. Sauté until softened.

5. Stir in diced tomatoes, tomato sauce, ground cinnamon, and ground nutmeg. Simmer for 10 minutes.

6. In a separate pot, melt butter over medium heat. Stir in flour and cook for 1 minute.

7. Gradually add milk, stirring constantly until thickened. Remove from heat and stir in grated Parmesan cheese.

8. In a baking dish, layer half of the eggplant slices, followed by the meat sauce. Top with remaining eggplant slices.

9. Pour the cheese sauce over the top layer.

10. Bake in the preheated oven for 30-35 minutes until golden and bubbly.

11. Serve hot and enjoy the rich and comforting Greek Moussaka.

Nutritional Value (Approx. per serving): Calories: 500 | Protein: 30g | Fiber: 6g | Healthy Fats: 30g | Carbohydrates: 25g

German Schnitzel with Potato Salad

Prep Time: 20 minutes | **Cook Time:** 20 minutes | **Per Serving:** 1 serving

Ingredients:

For the Schnitzel:

- 1 pork cutlet, pounded thin
- 1/4 cup all-purpose flour
- 1 egg, beaten
- 1/4 cup breadcrumbs
- Salt and pepper, to taste
- 2 tablespoons vegetable oil

For the Potato Salad:

- 1 cup boiled potatoes, sliced
- 1/4 cup red onion, chopped
- 1/4 cup pickles, diced
- 2 tablespoons mayonnaise
- 1 tablespoon mustard
- 1 tablespoon vinegar
- Salt and pepper, to taste

Instructions:

1. Season pork cutlet with salt and pepper.
2. Dredge the cutlet in flour, dip in beaten egg, and coat with breadcrumbs.
3. Heat vegetable oil in a skillet over medium heat. Fry the cutlet until golden brown on both sides, about 3-4 minutes per side. Drain on paper towels.
4. In a bowl, mix together boiled potatoes, red onion, pickles, mayonnaise, mustard, vinegar, salt, and pepper.
5. Serve the schnitzel hot with potato salad on the side.
6. Enjoy the crispy and savory German Schnitzel with tangy Potato Salad.

Nutritional Value (Approx. per serving): Calories: 600 | Protein: 30g | Fiber: 5g | Healthy Fats: 30g | Carbohydrates: 45g

British Fish and Chips

Prep Time: 20 minutes | **Cook Time:** 20 minutes | **Per Serving:** 1 serving

Ingredients:

- 1 fillet of white fish (e.g., cod or haddock)
- 1/4 cup all-purpose flour
- 1/4 cup beer or sparkling water
- 1 large potato, cut into fries
- Salt and pepper, to taste
- Vegetable oil, for frying
- Malt vinegar, for serving

Instructions:

1. Heat vegetable oil in a deep fryer or large pot to 350°F (175°C).
2. In a bowl, mix flour, beer or sparkling water, salt, and pepper to form a batter.
3. Dip the fish fillet into the batter, coating it evenly.
4. Fry the fish in the hot oil until golden brown and crispy, about 4-5 minutes. Drain on paper towels.
5. Fry the potato fries until golden and crispy, about 5-6 minutes. Drain on paper towels and season with salt.
6. Serve the fish and chips hot with a sprinkle of malt vinegar.
7. Enjoy the traditional and delicious British Fish and Chips.

Nutritional Value (Approx. per serving): Calories: 700 | Protein: 35g | Fiber: 5g | Healthy Fats: 30g | Carbohydrates: 70g

Swedish Meatballs with Lingonberry Sauce

Prep Time: 20 minutes | **Cook Time:** 20 minutes | **Per Serving:** 1 serving

Ingredients:

For the Meatballs:

- 4 oz ground beef
- 2 oz ground pork
- 1/4 cup breadcrumbs
- 1/4 cup milk
- 1/4 onion, grated
- 1 egg, beaten
- Salt and pepper, to taste
- 1/4 teaspoon allspice
- 1 tablespoon butter

For the Lingonberry Sauce:

- 1/4 cup lingonberry jam
- 2 tablespoons water

Instructions:

1. In a bowl, combine breadcrumbs and milk. Let it sit for a few minutes until the milk is absorbed.

2. Mix in ground beef, ground pork, grated onion, beaten egg, salt, pepper, and allspice.

3. Form the mixture into small meatballs.

4. Heat butter in a skillet over medium heat. Cook the meatballs until browned and cooked through, about 10-12 minutes. Remove and set aside.

5. In a small saucepan, combine lingonberry jam and water. Heat until the jam is melted and the sauce is smooth.

6. Serve the meatballs hot with lingonberry sauce on the side.

7. Enjoy the tender and flavorful Swedish Meatballs with sweet and tangy Lingonberry Sauce.

Nutritional Value (Approx. per serving): Calories: 450 | Protein: 25g | Fiber: 2g | Healthy Fats: 25g | Carbohydrates: 25g

Portuguese Grilled Sardines

Prep Time: 10 minutes | **Cook Time:** 10 minutes | **Per Serving:** 1 serving

Ingredients:

- 2 sardines, cleaned and gutted
- 1 tablespoon olive oil
- 1 clove garlic, minced
- 1 tablespoon lemon juice
- 1 tablespoon fresh parsley, chopped
- Salt and pepper, to taste

Instructions:

1. Preheat the grill to medium-high heat.
2. In a small bowl, mix olive oil, minced garlic, lemon juice, salt, and pepper.
3. Brush the sardines with the olive oil mixture.
4. Grill the sardines for 4-5 minutes on each side until cooked through and slightly charred.
5. Sprinkle with fresh parsley.
6. Serve hot and enjoy the simple and delicious Portuguese Grilled Sardines.

Nutritional Value (Approx. per serving): Calories: 250 | Protein: 25g | Fiber: 1g | Healthy Fats: 15g | Carbohydrates: 2g

Thai Green Curry with Chicken

Prep Time: 15 minutes | **Cook Time:** 25 minutes | **Per Serving:** 1 serving

Ingredients:

- 4 oz chicken breast, sliced thin
- 1/2 cup coconut milk
- 2 tablespoons green curry paste
- 1/2 cup mixed vegetables (bell peppers, zucchini, carrots)
- 1/4 cup bamboo shoots, drained
- 1 tablespoon fish sauce
- 1 tablespoon brown sugar
- 1/4 cup fresh basil leaves
- 1 tablespoon vegetable oil
- 1/4 cup chicken broth

Instructions:

1. Heat vegetable oil in a pan over medium heat. Add green curry paste and stir-fry for 1-2 minutes until fragrant.
2. Add sliced chicken breast and cook until the chicken is no longer pink.
3. Pour in coconut milk and chicken broth. Bring to a simmer.
4. Add mixed vegetables and bamboo shoots. Cook for 5-7 minutes until vegetables are tender.
5. Stir in fish sauce and brown sugar. Cook for another 2 minutes.
6. Add fresh basil leaves and remove from heat.
7. Serve hot and enjoy the flavorful and aromatic Thai Green Curry with Chicken.

Nutritional Value (Approx. per serving): Calories: 350 | Protein: 25g | Fiber: 4g | Healthy Fats: 20g | Carbohydrates: 15g

Indian Chicken Tikka Masala

Prep Time: 20 minutes | **Cook Time:** 30 minutes | **Per Serving:** 1 serving

Ingredients:

- 4 oz chicken breast, cubed
- 1/4 cup plain yogurt
- 1 tablespoon tikka masala paste
- 1/4 cup heavy cream
- 1/4 cup tomato sauce
- 1/2 onion, chopped
- 1 clove garlic, minced
- 1 teaspoon garam masala
- 1/2 teaspoon turmeric
- 1/2 teaspoon ground cumin
- 1 tablespoon vegetable oil
- Fresh cilantro, for garnish

Instructions:

1. In a bowl, mix cubed chicken breast with plain yogurt and tikka masala paste. Marinate for at least 30 minutes.

2. Heat vegetable oil in a pan over medium heat. Add chopped onion and minced garlic. Sauté until softened.

3. Add marinated chicken and cook until the chicken is no longer pink.

4. Stir in tomato sauce, garam masala, turmeric, and ground cumin. Cook for 5-7 minutes.

5. Pour in heavy cream and simmer for another 5 minutes until the sauce thickens.

6. Garnish with fresh cilantro.

7. Serve hot and enjoy the rich and creamy Indian Chicken Tikka Masala.

Nutritional Value (Approx. per serving): Calories: 400 | Protein: 30g | Fiber: 2g | Healthy Fats: 25g | Carbohydrates: 10g

Japanese Sushi Rolls (Maki)

Prep Time: 30 minutes | **Cook Time:** 10 minutes | **Per Serving:** 1 serving

Ingredients:

- 1/2 cup sushi rice
- 1/2 tablespoon rice vinegar
- 1/2 teaspoon sugar
- 1/4 teaspoon salt
- 1 nori sheet
- 1/4 cucumber, julienned
- 1/4 avocado, sliced
- 2 oz raw fish (tuna, salmon), sliced thin
- Soy sauce, for dipping
- Pickled ginger and wasabi, for serving

Instructions:

1. Cook sushi rice according to package instructions. Let it cool slightly.
2. In a small bowl, mix rice vinegar, sugar, and salt until dissolved. Stir into the cooked rice.
3. Place a nori sheet on a bamboo sushi mat. Spread an even layer of sushi rice over the nori, leaving a 1-inch border at the top.
4. Arrange cucumber, avocado, and raw fish slices in a line across the center of the rice.
5. Roll the sushi tightly using the bamboo mat, sealing the edge with a little water.
6. Slice the roll into bite-sized pieces with a sharp knife.
7. Serve with soy sauce, pickled ginger, and wasabi.
8. Enjoy the fresh and delicious Japanese Sushi Rolls (Maki).

Nutritional Value (Approx. per serving): Calories: 300 | Protein: 20g | Fiber: 4g | Healthy Fats: 10g | Carbohydrates: 35g

Mexican Chicken Mole

Prep Time: 20 minutes | **Cook Time:** 1 hour | **Per Serving:** 1 serving

Ingredients:

- 4 oz chicken breast
- 1/4 cup mole sauce (store-bought or homemade)
- 1/2 onion, chopped
- 1 clove garlic, minced
- 1/2 teaspoon ground cumin
- 1/2 teaspoon ground cinnamon
- 1/4 cup chicken broth
- 1 tablespoon vegetable oil
- Fresh cilantro, for garnish

Instructions:

1. Heat vegetable oil in a pan over medium heat. Add chopped onion and minced garlic. Sauté until softened.
2. Add chicken breast and cook until browned on both sides.
3. Stir in ground cumin and ground cinnamon. Cook for 1 minute.
4. Pour in chicken broth and mole sauce. Bring to a simmer.
5. Reduce heat to low, cover, and cook for 30-40 minutes until chicken is tender and sauce thickens.
6. Garnish with fresh cilantro.
7. Serve hot and enjoy the rich and complex flavors of Mexican Chicken Mole.

Nutritional Value (Approx. per serving): Calories: 400 | Protein: 25g | Fiber: 3g | Healthy Fats: 20g | Carbohydrates: 25g

Moroccan Lamb Tagine

Prep Time: 20 minutes | **Cook Time:** 2 hours | **Per Serving:** 1 serving

Ingredients:

- 4 oz lamb shoulder, cubed
- 1/2 onion, chopped
- 1 clove garlic, minced
- 1/2 cup diced tomatoes
- 1/2 cup chicken broth
- 1/4 cup dried apricots, chopped
- 1/4 cup chickpeas, drained and rinsed
- 1/2 teaspoon ground cumin
- 1/2 teaspoon ground cinnamon
- 1/4 teaspoon ground ginger
- 1 tablespoon olive oil
- Fresh cilantro, for garnish

Instructions:

1. Heat olive oil in a tagine or heavy-bottomed pot over medium heat. Add chopped onion and minced garlic. Sauté until softened.
2. Add lamb cubes and brown on all sides.
3. Stir in ground cumin, ground cinnamon, and ground ginger. Cook for 1 minute.
4. Add diced tomatoes, chicken broth, dried apricots, and chickpeas. Bring to a simmer.
5. Cover and reduce heat to low. Cook for 1.5-2 hours until lamb is tender.
6. Garnish with fresh cilantro.
7. Serve hot and enjoy the aromatic and flavorful Moroccan Lamb Tagine.

Nutritional Value (Approx. per serving): Calories: 450 | Protein: 30g | Fiber: 5g | Healthy Fats: 25g | Carbohydrates: 30g

Lebanese Falafel with Hummus

Prep Time: 30 minutes | **Cook Time:** 10 minutes | **Per Serving:** 1 serving

Ingredients:

For the Falafel:

- 1/2 cup chickpeas, soaked overnight and drained
- 1/4 onion, chopped
- 1 clove garlic, minced
- 1/4 cup fresh parsley
- 1/4 teaspoon ground cumin
- 1/4 teaspoon ground coriander
- Salt and pepper, to taste
- 1 tablespoon flour
- Vegetable oil, for frying

For the Hummus:

- 1/4 cup chickpeas, drained and rinsed
- 1 tablespoon tahini
- 1 tablespoon lemon juice
- 1 clove garlic, minced
- 1 tablespoon olive oil
- Salt, to taste

Instructions:

1. In a food processor, combine chickpeas, chopped onion, minced garlic, fresh parsley, ground cumin, ground coriander, salt, and pepper. Pulse until the mixture is coarse.

2. Add flour and pulse until the mixture comes together.

3. Form the mixture into small balls.

4. Heat vegetable oil in a skillet over medium heat. Fry the falafel balls until golden brown, about 3-4 minutes per side. Drain on paper towels.

5. In a food processor, blend chickpeas, tahini, lemon juice, minced garlic, olive oil, and salt until smooth.

6. Serve the falafel hot with hummus on the side.

7. Enjoy the crispy and flavorful Lebanese Falafel with creamy Hummus.

Nutritional Value (Approx. per serving): Calories: 350 | Protein: 15g | Fiber: 10g | Healthy Fats: 20g | Carbohydrates: 30g

Brazilian Feijoada

Prep Time: 20 minutes | **Cook Time:** 2 hours | **Per Serving:** 1 serving

Ingredients:

- 4 oz black beans, soaked overnight and drained
- 2 oz pork shoulder, cubed
- 2 oz chorizo sausage, sliced
- 1/2 onion, chopped
- 1 clove garlic, minced
- 1/2 tomato, chopped
- 1/2 cup chicken broth
- 1/2 teaspoon ground cumin
- 1/4 teaspoon ground paprika
- 1 bay leaf
- 1 tablespoon vegetable oil
- Fresh parsley, for garnish

Instructions:

1. Heat vegetable oil in a large pot over medium heat. Add chopped onion and minced garlic. Sauté until softened.
2. Add pork shoulder and chorizo sausage. Brown on all sides.
3. Stir in ground cumin, ground paprika, and bay leaf. Cook for 1 minute.
4. Add chopped tomato, black beans, and chicken broth. Bring to a boil.
5. Reduce heat to low, cover, and simmer for 1.5-2 hours until beans are tender and the stew thickens.
6. Garnish with fresh parsley.
7. Serve hot and enjoy the hearty and savory Brazilian Feijoada.

Nutritional Value (Approx. per serving): Calories: 500 | Protein: 30g | Fiber: 10g | Healthy Fats: 25g | Carbohydrates: 40g

Vietnamese Pho

Prep Time: 20 minutes | **Cook Time:** 30 minutes | **Per Serving:** 1 serving

Ingredients:

- 4 oz rice noodles
- 4 oz beef sirloin, thinly sliced
- 4 cups beef broth
- 1/2 onion, thinly sliced
- 1 clove garlic, minced
- 1/2 teaspoon ground ginger
- 1 tablespoon fish sauce
- 1 star anise
- Fresh basil, cilantro, and mint, for garnish
- Bean sprouts, for serving
- Lime wedges, for serving
- Sriracha and hoisin sauce, for serving

Instructions:

1. In a large pot, bring beef broth to a boil. Add thinly sliced onion, minced garlic, ground ginger, fish sauce, and star anise. Simmer for 20 minutes.

2. Cook rice noodles according to package instructions. Drain and set aside.

3. Arrange thinly sliced beef sirloin in serving bowls.

4. Pour hot broth over the beef to cook it.

5. Add cooked rice noodles to the bowls.

6. Garnish with fresh basil, cilantro, mint, and bean sprouts.

7. Serve with lime wedges, sriracha, and hoisin sauce.

8. Enjoy the aromatic and comforting Vietnamese Pho.

Nutritional Value (Approx. per serving): Calories: 400 | Protein: 25g | Fiber: 5g | Healthy Fats: 10g | Carbohydrates: 60g

28-Day Meal Plan for Gut Health

Week 1

Day 1:

- **Breakfast:** Smoothie with Spinach and Berries
- **Lunch:** Grilled Chicken Salad with Mixed Greens
- **Dinner:** Roasted Salmon with Asparagus and Lemon
- **Snack:** Greek Yogurt with Honey and Walnuts

Day 2:

- **Breakfast:** Chia Seed Pudding
- **Lunch:** Quinoa and Black Bean Stuffed Bell Peppers
- **Dinner:** Vegetable Stir-Fry with Tofu
- **Snack:** Carrot and Hummus Sticks

Day 3:

- **Breakfast:** Avocado Toast
- **Lunch:** Lentil Soup with Kale and Carrots
- **Dinner:** Quinoa and Kale Stuffed Portobello Mushrooms
- **Snack:** Apple Slices with Almond Butter

Day 4:

- **Breakfast:** Greek Yogurt Parfait
- **Lunch:** Salmon and Avocado Wrap with Whole Grain Tortilla
- **Dinner:** Grilled Chicken with Quinoa Salad
- **Snack:** Mixed Nuts and Seeds

Day 5:

- **Breakfast:** Oatmeal with Berries and Almonds
- **Lunch:** Mediterranean Chickpea Salad

- **Dinner:** Chickpea and Spinach Curry
- **Snack:** Fresh Fruit Salad

Day 6:

- **Breakfast:** Quinoa Breakfast Bowl
- **Lunch:** Turkey and Vegetable Stir-Fry with Brown Rice
- **Dinner:** Turkey Meatballs with Zucchini Noodles
- **Snack:** Celery Sticks with Peanut Butter

Day 7:

- **Breakfast:** Blueberry Buckwheat Pancakes
- **Lunch:** Sweet Potato and Black Bean Tacos with Cilantro Lime Slaw
- **Dinner:** Baked Cod with Garlic and Herbs
- **Snack:** Dark Chocolate Squares

Week 2

Day 8:

- **Breakfast:** Spinach and Mushroom Egg White Omelette
- **Lunch:** Buddha Bowl with Roasted Vegetables and Tahini Dressing
- **Dinner:** Vegetarian Chili with Beans and Sweet Potatoes
- **Snack:** Kale Chips

Day 9:

- **Breakfast:** Green Revitalizer Smoothie
- **Lunch:** Classic Cobb Salad
- **Dinner:** Moroccan Lamb Tagine
- **Snack:** Cottage Cheese with Pineapple

Day 10:

- **Breakfast:** Overnight Oats with Chia Seeds
- **Lunch:** Barbecue Pulled Pork Sandwiches
- **Dinner:** Lebanese Falafel with Hummus

- **Snack:** Edamame

Day 11:

- **Breakfast:** Smoothie with Spinach and Berries
- **Lunch:** New England Clam Chowder
- **Dinner:** Brazilian Feijoada
- **Snack:** Roasted Chickpeas

Day 12:

- **Breakfast:** Chia Seed Pudding
- **Lunch:** Southern Shrimp and Grits
- **Dinner:** Vietnamese Pho
- **Snack:** Cucumber Slices with Tzatziki

Day 13:

- **Breakfast:** Avocado Toast
- **Lunch:** California Turkey Avocado Wrap
- **Dinner:** Thai Green Curry with Chicken
- **Snack:** Popcorn

Day 14:

- **Breakfast:** Greek Yogurt Parfait
- **Lunch:** Tex-Mex Chicken Enchiladas
- **Dinner:** Indian Chicken Tikka Masala
- **Snack:** Frozen Grapes

Week 3

Day 15:

- **Breakfast:** Oatmeal with Berries and Almonds
- **Lunch:** Midwest Beef Pot Roast
- **Dinner:** Japanese Sushi Rolls (Maki)
- **Snack:** Almonds

Day 16:

- **Breakfast:** Quinoa Breakfast Bowl
- **Lunch:** Buttermilk Fried Chicken
- **Dinner:** Mexican Chicken Mole
- **Snack:** Bell Pepper Strips

Day 17:

- **Breakfast:** Blueberry Buckwheat Pancakes
- **Lunch:** Italian Caprese Salad
- **Dinner:** Moroccan Lamb Tagine
- **Snack:** Yogurt with Berries

Day 18:

- **Breakfast:** Spinach and Mushroom Egg White Omelette
- **Lunch:** French Coq au Vin
- **Dinner:** Lebanese Falafel with Hummus
- **Snack:** Trail Mix

Day 19:

- **Breakfast:** Green Revitalizer Smoothie
- **Lunch:** Spanish Paella
- **Dinner:** Brazilian Feijoada
- **Snack:** Sliced Oranges

Day 20:

- **Breakfast:** Overnight Oats with Chia Seeds
- **Lunch:** Greek Moussaka
- **Dinner:** Vietnamese Pho
- **Snack:** Avocado Slices

Day 21:

- **Breakfast:** Smoothie with Spinach and Berries
- **Lunch:** German Schnitzel with Potato Salad
- **Dinner:** Thai Green Curry with Chicken
- **Snack:** Carrot Sticks with Hummus

Week 4

Day 22:

- **Breakfast:** Chia Seed Pudding
- **Lunch:** British Fish and Chips
- **Dinner:** Indian Chicken Tikka Masala
- **Snack:** Dried Fruit

Day 23:

- **Breakfast:** Avocado Toast
- **Lunch:** Swedish Meatballs with Lingonberry Sauce
- **Dinner:** Japanese Sushi Rolls (Maki)
- **Snack:** Cherry Tomatoes

Day 24:

- **Breakfast:** Greek Yogurt Parfait
- **Lunch:** Portuguese Grilled Sardines
- **Dinner:** Mexican Chicken Mole
- **Snack:** Rice Cakes with Nut Butter

Day 25:

- **Breakfast:** Oatmeal with Berries and Almonds
- **Lunch:** Classic Cobb Salad
- **Dinner:** Moroccan Lamb Tagine
- **Snack:** Apple Slices

Day 26:

- **Breakfast:** Quinoa Breakfast Bowl
- **Lunch:** Barbecue Pulled Pork Sandwiches
- **Dinner:** Lebanese Falafel with Hummus
- **Snack:** Roasted Almonds

Day 27:

- **Breakfast:** Blueberry Buckwheat Pancakes
- **Lunch:** New England Clam Chowder
- **Dinner:** Brazilian Feijoada
- **Snack:** Dark Chocolate Squares

Day 28:

- **Breakfast:** Spinach and Mushroom Egg White Omelette
- **Lunch:** Southern Shrimp and Grits
- **Dinner:** Vietnamese Pho
- **Snack:** Mixed Berries

Chapter 11: Special Diets for Gut Health

Gluten-Free

Understanding a Gluten-Free Diet

A gluten-free diet excludes all forms of gluten, a protein found in wheat, barley, rye, and their derivatives. This diet is essential for individuals with celiac disease, non-celiac gluten sensitivity, and wheat allergies. Adopting a gluten-free diet can also benefit those seeking to improve digestive health and reduce inflammation.

Benefits of a Gluten-Free Diet

1. **Alleviates Digestive Symptoms:**

    o Reduces bloating, gas, diarrhea, and constipation in individuals with gluten intolerance or sensitivity.

2. **Enhances Nutrient Absorption:**

    o Improves nutrient absorption in individuals with celiac disease by healing intestinal damage caused by gluten.

3. **Reduces Inflammation:**

    o Lowers systemic inflammation, benefiting those with autoimmune conditions and chronic inflammation.

4. **Boosts Energy Levels:**

    o Prevents energy crashes and promotes consistent energy levels throughout the day.

5. **Improves Overall Well-being:**

    o Enhances mood, mental clarity, and general well-being by eliminating gluten-related discomfort.

Foods to Include and Avoid

Include:

1. **Whole Grains:**

    o **Rice:** Brown rice, white rice, wild rice.

    o **Quinoa:** High in protein and fiber.

- o **Buckwheat:** Despite its name, it is gluten-free.
- o **Amaranth:** Nutritious and versatile.

2. **Legumes:**
   - o Beans, lentils, chickpeas, and peas.

3. **Fruits and Vegetables:**
   - o All fresh fruits and vegetables are naturally gluten-free.

4. **Nuts and Seeds:**
   - o Almonds, chia seeds, flaxseeds, sunflower seeds.

5. **Gluten-Free Flours:**
   - o Almond flour, coconut flour, rice flour, tapioca flour, and sorghum flour.

6. **Protein Sources:**
   - o Meat, poultry, fish, seafood, tofu, and tempeh (ensure no gluten-containing marinades or sauces).

7. **Dairy and Dairy Alternatives:**
   - o Milk, cheese, yogurt, and plant-based alternatives like almond milk, coconut milk, and soy milk.

Avoid:

1. **Wheat Products:**
   - o Bread, pasta, cereals, pastries, and other baked goods made from wheat.

2. **Barley and Rye:**
   - o Foods containing barley or rye, such as certain beers and malt products.

3. **Processed Foods:**
   - o Many processed foods contain hidden gluten, including soups, sauces, dressings, and processed meats.

4. **Certain Condiments:**
   - o Soy sauce (unless labeled gluten-free), malt vinegar, and some salad dressings.

5. **Baked Goods:**

   o Cakes, cookies, muffins, and other pastries made with gluten-containing flour.

Practical Tips for a Gluten-Free Lifestyle

1. **Meal Planning:**

   o Plan meals ahead to ensure they are balanced and gluten-free. Use fresh, whole ingredients to avoid hidden gluten.

2. **Reading Labels:**

   o Carefully read food labels to check for gluten-containing ingredients. Look for certified gluten-free labels.

3. **Cooking at Home:**

   o Cooking at home allows you to control ingredients and avoid cross-contamination. Experiment with gluten-free grains and flours.

4. **Restaurant Dining:**

   o When dining out, communicate your dietary needs clearly to the restaurant staff. Choose restaurants that offer gluten-free options.

5. **Gluten-Free Snacks:**

   o Keep snacks like fresh fruits, nuts, seeds, gluten-free crackers, and dairy-free yogurt on hand for quick and safe options.

6. **Cross-Contamination Prevention:**

   o Use separate kitchen utensils, cutting boards, and appliances for gluten-free cooking to avoid cross-contamination.

Sample Meal Ideas

Breakfast:

- **Gluten-Free Smoothie:**

   o Blend almond milk, spinach, blueberries, chia seeds, and a small banana.

- **Quinoa Porridge:**

   o Cook quinoa with almond milk, and top with strawberries and a drizzle of maple syrup.

Lunch:

- **Grilled Chicken Salad:**

  - Mixed greens with grilled chicken, cherry tomatoes, cucumber, carrots, and a gluten-free dressing.

- **Stuffed Bell Peppers:**

  - Bell peppers stuffed with quinoa, spinach, and ground turkey.

Dinner:

- **Baked Salmon:**

  - Baked salmon with a side of roasted carrots and quinoa.

- **Stir-Fried Vegetables:**

  - Stir-fry zucchini, bell peppers, and spinach with tofu and gluten-free soy sauce.

Snacks:

- **Dairy-Free Yogurt with Berries:**

  - Coconut yogurt topped with blueberries and chia seeds.

- **Gluten-Free Crackers with Almond Butter:**

  - Gluten-free rice crackers spread with almond butter.

Dairy-Free

Understanding a Dairy-Free Diet

A dairy-free diet excludes all forms of dairy products, including milk, cheese, butter, and yogurt. This diet is necessary for individuals with lactose intolerance, milk allergies, or a preference for plant-based diets. Adopting a dairy-free diet can also benefit those seeking to improve digestive health and reduce inflammation.

Benefits of a Dairy-Free Diet

1. **Alleviates Digestive Symptoms:**
   - Reduces bloating, gas, diarrhea, and stomach cramps in individuals with lactose intolerance or milk allergies.

2. **Enhances Nutrient Absorption:**
   - Improves nutrient absorption by minimizing gut irritation caused by dairy products.

3. **Reduces Inflammation:**
   - Lowers systemic inflammation, benefiting those with autoimmune conditions and chronic inflammation.

4. **Improves Skin Health:**
   - May reduce acne and other skin conditions related to dairy consumption.

5. **Supports Weight Management:**
   - Helps with weight management by reducing calorie and saturated fat intake from dairy products.

Foods to Include and Avoid

Include:

1. **Plant-Based Milks:**
   - **Almond Milk:** Low in calories and rich in vitamin E.
   - **Coconut Milk:** Creamy texture, good for cooking and baking.
   - **Soy Milk:** High in protein and calcium-fortified.
   - **Oat Milk:** Creamy, with a mild flavor, often fortified with vitamins.

2. **Dairy-Free Yogurts:**
   - **Coconut Yogurt:** Rich and creamy, good for probiotics.

- **Almond Yogurt:** Light and nutty, often fortified with calcium.
- **Soy Yogurt:** High in protein and similar in texture to dairy yogurt.

3. **Dairy-Free Cheeses:**
    - **Nut-Based Cheeses:** Made from cashews, almonds, or other nuts.
    - **Soy Cheese:** Made from soy protein, often fortified with calcium.
    - **Coconut Cheese:** Made from coconut oil and starches, good for melting.

4. **Fruits and Vegetables:**
    - All fresh fruits and vegetables are naturally dairy-free.

5. **Nuts and Seeds:**
    - Almonds, cashews, chia seeds, flaxseeds, and sunflower seeds.

6. **Whole Grains:**
    - Rice, quinoa, millet, buckwheat, and oats (ensure they are gluten-free if needed).

7. **Protein Sources:**
    - Meat, poultry, fish, seafood, tofu, tempeh, and legumes.

Avoid:

1. **Milk:**
    - Cow's milk, goat's milk, and other animal milks.

2. **Cheese:**
    - All types of cheese made from animal milk.

3. **Butter and Cream:**
    - All dairy-based butters and creams.

4. **Yogurt:**
    - Traditional cow's milk or goat's milk yogurt.

5. **Processed Foods:**
    - Many processed foods contain hidden dairy, such as baked goods, sauces, and processed meats.

Practical Tips for a Dairy-Free Lifestyle

1. **Meal Planning:**

   o Plan meals ahead to ensure they are balanced and dairy-free. Use fresh, whole ingredients to avoid hidden dairy.

2. **Reading Labels:**

   o Carefully read food labels to check for dairy-containing ingredients. Look for certified dairy-free labels.

3. **Cooking at Home:**

   o Cooking at home allows you to control ingredients and avoid cross-contamination. Experiment with dairy-free substitutes for milk, cheese, and yogurt.

4. **Restaurant Dining:**

   o When dining out, communicate your dietary needs clearly to the restaurant staff. Choose restaurants that offer dairy-free options.

5. **Dairy-Free Snacks:**

   o Keep snacks like fresh fruits, nuts, seeds, gluten-free crackers, and dairy-free yogurt on hand for quick and safe options.

6. **Baking Dairy-Free:**

   o Substitute dairy milk with plant-based milks, butter with coconut oil or dairy-free margarine, and use dairy-free yogurt in recipes.

Sample Meal Ideas

Breakfast:

- **Dairy-Free Smoothie:**

  o Blend almond milk, spinach, blueberries, chia seeds, and a small banana.

- **Overnight Oats:**

  o Combine oats with coconut milk, chia seeds, and strawberries, and refrigerate overnight.

Lunch:

- **Quinoa Salad:**

  o Mixed greens with quinoa, cherry tomatoes, cucumber, avocado, and a lemon vinaigrette.

- **Vegetable Stir-Fry:**
  - Stir-fry broccoli, bell peppers, snap peas, and tofu with coconut aminos.

Dinner:

- **Baked Salmon:**
  - Baked salmon with a side of roasted carrots and quinoa.
- **Stuffed Bell Peppers:**
  - Bell peppers stuffed with quinoa, spinach, and ground turkey.

Snacks:

- **Dairy-Free Yogurt with Berries:**
  - Coconut yogurt topped with blueberries and chia seeds.
- **Gluten-Free Crackers with Hummus:**
  - Gluten-free rice crackers served with homemade hummus

Low-FODMAP

Understanding a Low-FODMAP Diet

A low-FODMAP diet restricts foods high in fermentable oligosaccharides, disaccharides, monosaccharides, and polyols (FODMAPs). These short-chain carbohydrates can be poorly absorbed in the small intestine, leading to digestive distress in individuals with irritable bowel syndrome (IBS) and other functional gastrointestinal disorders. The low-FODMAP diet is designed to alleviate symptoms such as bloating, gas, diarrhea, and constipation by reducing the intake of these problematic carbohydrates.

Benefits of a Low-FODMAP Diet

1. **Alleviates Digestive Symptoms:**

    o Reduces bloating, gas, diarrhea, and constipation in individuals with IBS or other digestive disorders.

2. **Improves Quality of Life:**

    o Enhances overall well-being by reducing gastrointestinal discomfort and improving daily functioning.

3. **Supports Gut Health:**

    o Helps balance the gut microbiome by minimizing foods that can cause dysbiosis (microbial imbalance).

4. **Personalized Approach:**

    o The diet involves a reintroduction phase, allowing individuals to identify specific triggers and tailor their diet accordingly.

5. **Scientific Backing:**

    o Numerous studies have demonstrated the effectiveness of the low-FODMAP diet in managing IBS symptoms.

Foods to Include and Avoid

Include:

1. **Low-FODMAP Fruits:**

    o **Bananas:** Ripe but not overripe.

    o **Blueberries:** In moderation.

    o **Strawberries:** Fresh or frozen.

    o **Oranges:** Whole or as juice (in small amounts).

2. **Low-FODMAP Vegetables:**

   o **Carrots:** Raw or cooked.

   o **Spinach:** Fresh or cooked.

   o **Zucchini:** Fresh or cooked.

   o **Bell Peppers:** All colors.

3. **Proteins:**

   o **Eggs:** Cooked in various ways.

   o **Chicken:** Fresh and cooked without high-FODMAP seasonings.

   o **Fish and Seafood:** Fresh or canned in water.

   o **Tofu:** Firm or extra-firm, plain.

4. **Grains:**

   o **Rice:** White, brown, or wild.

   o **Quinoa:** Cooked plain.

   o **Oats:** Rolled or quick oats (ensure gluten-free if needed).

5. **Nuts and Seeds:**

   o **Almonds:** In small amounts.

   o **Peanuts:** Plain, unsalted.

   o **Chia Seeds:** Great for adding to smoothies or yogurt.

   o **Pumpkin Seeds:** Plain, unsalted.

6. **Dairy Alternatives:**

   o **Lactose-Free Milk:** Cow's milk without lactose.

   o **Almond Milk:** Unsweetened.

   o **Coconut Milk:** Limited to ½ cup per serving.

Avoid:

1. **High-FODMAP Fruits:**

   o **Apples:** Fresh, dried, or juiced.

   o **Pears:** All varieties.

- o **Mangoes:** Fresh or dried.
- o **Cherries:** Fresh, dried, or juiced.

2. **High-FODMAP Vegetables:**
   - o **Onions:** All types.
   - o **Garlic:** Fresh or powdered.
   - o **Cauliflower:** Fresh or cooked.
   - o **Mushrooms:** All varieties.

3. **Legumes:**
   - o **Beans:** Kidney beans, black beans, and others.
   - o **Lentils:** Unless canned and thoroughly rinsed.
   - o **Chickpeas:** Fresh or dried.

4. **Dairy:**
   - o **Milk:** Cow's milk, goat's milk, and other high-lactose dairy products.
   - o **Yogurt:** Regular cow's milk yogurt.
   - o **Soft Cheeses:** Brie, ricotta, and cream cheese.

5. **Sweeteners:**
   - o **High-Fructose Corn Syrup:** Found in many processed foods.
   - o **Honey:** High in fructose.
   - o **Agave Nectar:** High in fructose.

6. **Certain Grains:**
   - o **Wheat:** Bread, pasta, cereals, and pastries.
   - o **Rye:** Bread and other products.
   - o **Barley:** Found in soups and some processed foods.

Practical Tips for a Low-FODMAP Lifestyle

1. **Meal Planning:**

   - Plan meals ahead to ensure they are balanced and low-FODMAP. Use fresh,

   - whole ingredients to avoid hidden FODMAPs.

2. **Reading Labels:**

   - Carefully read food labels to check for high-FODMAP ingredients. Look for certified low-FODMAP products when available.

3. **Cooking at Home:**

   - Cooking at home allows you to control ingredients and avoid cross-contamination. Use low-FODMAP seasonings like ginger, turmeric, and chives instead of garlic and onions.

4. **Restaurant Dining:**

   - When dining out, communicate your dietary needs clearly to the restaurant staff. Choose restaurants that offer low-FODMAP options or customizable dishes.

5. **Low-FODMAP Snacks:**

   - Keep snacks like fresh fruits, nuts, seeds, gluten-free crackers, and lactose-free yogurt on hand for quick and safe options.

6. **Hydration:**

   - Drink plenty of water and avoid high-FODMAP beverages like certain fruit juices and sweetened drinks.

Sample Meal Ideas

Breakfast:

- **Low-FODMAP Smoothie:**
  - Blend lactose-free milk, spinach, blueberries, chia seeds, and a small banana.

- **Overnight Oats:**
  - Combine oats with lactose-free milk, chia seeds, and strawberries, and refrigerate overnight.

Lunch:

- **Grilled Chicken Salad:**
  - Mixed greens with grilled chicken, cherry tomatoes, cucumber, carrots, and a low-FODMAP dressing.

- **Stuffed Bell Peppers:**
  - Bell peppers stuffed with quinoa, spinach, and ground turkey.

Dinner:

- **Baked Salmon:**
  - Baked salmon with a side of roasted carrots and quinoa.

- **Stir-Fried Vegetables:**
  - Stir-fry zucchini, bell peppers, and spinach with tofu and a low-FODMAP soy sauce.

Snacks:

- **Lactose-Free Yogurt with Berries:**
  - Lactose-free yogurt topped with blueberries and chia seeds.

- **Gluten-Free Crackers with Almond Butter:**
  - Gluten-free rice crackers spread with almond butter.

Plant-Based Diets

Understanding a Plant-Based Diet

A plant-based diet focuses on foods primarily from plants. This includes not only fruits and vegetables, but also nuts, seeds, oils, whole grains, legumes, and beans. While it doesn't mean that you are vegetarian or vegan and entirely give up meat or animal products, you are proportionately choosing more of your foods from plant sources.

Benefits of a Plant-Based Diet

1. **Improves Digestive Health:**

   o High in fiber, which promotes healthy digestion and regular bowel movements.

2. **Reduces Inflammation:**

   o Rich in antioxidants and phytonutrients that help reduce inflammation.

3. **Supports Weight Management:**

   o Typically lower in calories and higher in nutrients, which can help with weight loss or maintenance.

4. **Lowers Risk of Chronic Diseases:**

   o Associated with a reduced risk of heart disease, diabetes, and certain cancers.

5. **Boosts Energy Levels:**

   o Provides steady energy from whole foods without the crashes associated with processed foods.

Foods to Include and Avoid

Include:

1. **Fruits:**

   o Apples, bananas, berries, oranges, and grapes.

   o Exotic fruits like mangoes, papayas, and kiwis.

2. **Vegetables:**

   o Leafy greens such as spinach, kale, and Swiss chard.

   o Cruciferous vegetables like broccoli, cauliflower, and Brussels sprouts.

   o Root vegetables like carrots, beets, and sweet potatoes.

3. **Whole Grains:**
    - Quinoa, brown rice, oats, barley, and farro.
    - Whole grain bread, pasta, and cereals.

4. **Legumes:**
    - Beans, lentils, chickpeas, and peas.
    - Soy products like tofu, tempeh, and edamame.

5. **Nuts and Seeds:**
    - Almonds, walnuts, cashews, chia seeds, flaxseeds, and hemp seeds.
    - Nut butters like almond butter and peanut butter.

6. **Healthy Fats:**
    - Avocados, olive oil, coconut oil, and nut oils.

Avoid:

1. **Processed Foods:**
    - Foods with added sugars, refined grains, and artificial ingredients.
    - Pre-packaged meals and snacks high in unhealthy fats and sodium.

2. **Animal Products (for strict plant-based eaters):**
    - Meat, poultry, fish, dairy, and eggs.

3. **Refined Grains:**
    - White bread, white rice, and refined pasta.

4. **Sugary Beverages:**
    - Sodas, energy drinks, and sweetened teas.

5. **Junk Food:**
    - Chips, candy, cookies, and other highly processed snacks.

Practical Tips for a Plant-Based Lifestyle

1. **Meal Planning:**
    - Plan meals ahead to ensure they are balanced and plant-based. Focus on whole, minimally processed foods.

2. **Reading Labels:**

- Carefully read food labels to check for hidden animal products or excessive processing.

3. **Cooking at Home:**

   - Cooking at home allows you to control ingredients and experiment with plant-based recipes. Use herbs and spices to enhance flavors.

4. **Restaurant Dining:**

   - When dining out, communicate your dietary preferences clearly to the restaurant staff. Choose restaurants that offer plant-based options or customizable dishes.

5. **Plant-Based Snacks:**

   - Keep snacks like fresh fruits, nuts, seeds, hummus with veggies, and whole grain crackers on hand for quick and nutritious options.

6. **Transition Gradually:**

   - Start by incorporating more plant-based meals into your diet gradually. Replace animal products with plant-based alternatives over time.

Sample Meal Ideas

Breakfast:

- **Plant-Based Smoothie:**

  - Blend almond milk, spinach, banana, chia seeds, and a handful of berries.

- **Overnight Oats:**

  - Combine oats with almond milk, chia seeds, and your favorite fruits, and refrigerate overnight.

Lunch:

- **Quinoa Salad:**

  - Mixed greens with quinoa, chickpeas, cherry tomatoes, cucumber, avocado, and a lemon-tahini dressing.

- **Vegetable Stir-Fry:**

  - Stir-fry broccoli, bell peppers, snap peas, and tofu with coconut aminos over brown rice.

Dinner:

- **Lentil Soup:**
    - A hearty soup made with lentils, carrots, celery, onions, and tomatoes.
- **Stuffed Bell Peppers:**
    - Bell peppers stuffed with quinoa, black beans, corn, and topped with avocado.

Snacks:

- **Fruit and Nut Mix:**
    - A mix of dried fruits, nuts, and seeds.
- **Vegetable Sticks with Hummus:**
    - Carrot, celery, and bell pepper sticks with homemade hummus.

Chapter 12: Meal Planning and Preparation

Sample Weekly Plans

Week 1: Balanced Gut Health

Day 1:

- **Breakfast:** Plant-Based Smoothie with almond milk, spinach, banana, chia seeds, and berries.

- **Lunch:** Quinoa Salad with mixed greens, chickpeas, cherry tomatoes, cucumber, avocado, and lemon-tahini dressing.

- **Dinner:** Lentil Soup with carrots, celery, onions, and tomatoes.

- **Snack:** Apple slices with almond butter.

Day 2:

- **Breakfast:** Overnight Oats with almond milk, chia seeds, and blueberries.

- **Lunch:** Vegetable Stir-Fry with broccoli, bell peppers, snap peas, and tofu over brown rice.

- **Dinner:** Baked Salmon with roasted carrots and quinoa.

- **Snack:** Carrot sticks with hummus.

Day 3:

- **Breakfast:** Chia Pudding with coconut milk, chia seeds, and mango.

- **Lunch:** Stuffed Bell Peppers with quinoa, black beans, corn, and avocado.

- **Dinner:** Grilled Chicken Salad with mixed greens, cherry tomatoes, cucumber, carrots, and a low-FODMAP dressing.

- **Snack:** Mixed nuts and seeds.

Day 4:

- **Breakfast:** Smoothie Bowl with almond milk, spinach, banana, strawberries, and granola.

- **Lunch:** Quinoa and Black Bean Tacos with avocado, lettuce, and salsa.

- **Dinner:** Baked Cod with roasted sweet potatoes and steamed broccoli.

- **Snack:** Dairy-free yogurt with berries.

Day 5:

- **Breakfast:** Avocado Toast on gluten-free bread with a side of fresh fruit.
- **Lunch:** Lentil and Vegetable Soup with a side of gluten-free crackers.
- **Dinner:** Stir-Fried Tempeh with bell peppers, zucchini, and brown rice.
- **Snack:** Fresh berries and almond milk.

Day 6:

- **Breakfast:** Smoothie with coconut milk, kale, pineapple, and chia seeds.
- **Lunch:** Chickpea Salad Sandwich on gluten-free bread with lettuce, tomato, and avocado.
- **Dinner:** Grilled Shrimp Skewers with quinoa salad and steamed asparagus.
- **Snack:** Mixed fruit bowl.

Day 7:

- **Breakfast:** Dairy-Free Yogurt Parfait with granola, blueberries, and flaxseeds.
- **Lunch:** Stuffed Sweet Potatoes with black beans, corn, avocado, and a lime-cilantro dressing.
- **Dinner:** Baked Tofu with stir-fried vegetables and rice noodles.
- **Snack:** Apple slices with peanut butter.

Week 2: Focus on Probiotics and Prebiotics

Day 1:

- **Breakfast:** Kefir Smoothie with blueberries, spinach, and chia seeds.
- **Lunch:** Quinoa Salad with chickpeas, mixed greens, tomatoes, cucumber, and a probiotic-rich dressing.
- **Dinner:** Tempeh Stir-Fry with broccoli, bell peppers, and brown rice.
- **Snack:** Dairy-free yogurt with flaxseeds.

Day 2:

- **Breakfast:** Overnight Oats with almond milk, chia seeds, and probiotic-rich coconut yogurt.
- **Lunch:** Lentil Soup with carrots, celery, onions, and sauerkraut.
- **Dinner:** Grilled Salmon with roasted garlic asparagus and quinoa.
- **Snack:** Mixed nuts and seeds.

Day 3:

- **Breakfast:** Chia Pudding with coconut milk, chia seeds, and probiotic-rich berries.
- **Lunch:** Chickpea and Avocado Salad with a side of fermented vegetables.
- **Dinner:** Stuffed Bell Peppers with quinoa, black beans, and a side of kimchi.
- **Snack:** Fresh fruit and almond butter.

Day 4:

- **Breakfast:** Smoothie Bowl with kefir, spinach, banana, strawberries, and granola.
- **Lunch:** Quinoa and Black Bean Tacos with avocado, lettuce, salsa, and a side of probiotic-rich pickles.
- **Dinner:** Baked Cod with roasted sweet potatoes and a side of fermented vegetables.
- **Snack:** Mixed fruit bowl.

Day 5:

- **Breakfast:** Avocado Toast on gluten-free bread with a side of probiotic-rich kefir.
- **Lunch:** Lentil and Vegetable Soup with a side of sauerkraut.

- **Dinner:** Stir-Fried Tempeh with bell peppers, zucchini, and brown rice.
- **Snack:** Fresh berries and almond milk.

Day 6:

- **Breakfast:** Smoothie with coconut milk, kale, pineapple, chia seeds, and a probiotic supplement.
- **Lunch:** Chickpea Salad Sandwich on gluten-free bread with lettuce, tomato, avocado, and a side of fermented vegetables.
- **Dinner:** Grilled Shrimp Skewers with quinoa salad and steamed asparagus.
- **Snack:** Mixed fruit bowl.

Day 7:

- **Breakfast:** Dairy-Free Yogurt Parfait with granola, blueberries, flaxseeds, and a probiotic supplement.
- **Lunch:** Stuffed Sweet Potatoes with black beans, corn, avocado, and a lime-cilantro dressing.
- **Dinner:** Baked Tofu with stir-fried vegetables and rice noodles.
- **Snack:** Apple slices with peanut butter.

Tips for Creating Your Own Weekly Plan

1. **Balance Nutrients:**
   - Ensure each meal includes a balance of proteins, healthy fats, and carbohydrates.

2. **Variety:**
   - Rotate different fruits, vegetables, grains, and protein sources to get a wide range of nutrients.

3. **Preparation:**
   - Spend time on meal prep at the beginning of the week to make daily cooking easier.

4. **Listen to Your Body:**
   - Adjust portions and ingredients based on how your body responds.

5. **Stay Hydrated:**
   - Drink plenty of water and include hydrating foods like fruits and vegetables.

6. **Incorporate Fermented Foods:**
   - Add a variety of fermented foods like yogurt, kefir, sauerkraut, and kimchi to support gut health.

7. **Snack Smart:**
   - Keep healthy snacks on hand to avoid reaching for processed foods.

8. **Experiment with Recipes:**
   - Don't be afraid to try new recipes and ingredients to keep meals exciting and enjoyable.

9. **Include Probiotics and Prebiotics:**
   - Regularly incorporate foods that support a healthy gut microbiome, such as yogurt, kefir, sauerkraut, garlic, onions, and bananas.

10. **Mindful Eating:**
    - Practice mindful eating by savoring your meals, chewing thoroughly, and paying attention to hunger and fullness cues.

Sample Weekly Plan: Week 3 - Gut Healing Focus

Day 1:

- **Breakfast:** Smoothie with almond milk, spinach, banana, flaxseeds, and blueberries.

- **Lunch:** Quinoa Salad with chickpeas, mixed greens, cherry tomatoes, cucumber, and olive oil dressing.

- **Dinner:** Grilled Chicken Breast with roasted vegetables (carrots, zucchini, and bell peppers) and brown rice.

- **Snack:** Fresh fruit bowl with a mix of berries and apple slices.

Day 2:

- **Breakfast:** Overnight Oats with chia seeds, almond milk, and a dollop of dairy-free yogurt.

- **Lunch:** Lentil Soup with celery, carrots, onions, and a side of gluten-free bread.

- **Dinner:** Baked Salmon with a side of quinoa and steamed broccoli.

- **Snack:** Carrot sticks with hummus.

Day 3:

- **Breakfast:** Chia Pudding with coconut milk, chia seeds, and fresh mango.

- **Lunch:** Stuffed Bell Peppers with quinoa, black beans, corn, and a lime-cilantro dressing.

- **Dinner:** Vegetable Stir-Fry with tofu, bell peppers, broccoli, and brown rice.

- **Snack:** Mixed nuts and seeds.

Day 4:

- **Breakfast:** Smoothie Bowl with almond milk, kale, banana, strawberries, and granola.

- **Lunch:** Chickpea Salad with avocado, cucumber, tomatoes, and lemon-tahini dressing.

- **Dinner:** Baked Cod with roasted sweet potatoes and green beans.

- **Snack:** Fresh berries with almond milk.

Day 5:

- **Breakfast:** Avocado Toast on gluten-free bread with a side of mixed fruit.

- **Lunch:** Quinoa and Black Bean Tacos with avocado, lettuce, salsa, and a side of kimchi.
- **Dinner:** Grilled Tempeh with stir-fried vegetables and rice noodles.
- **Snack:** Dairy-free yogurt with blueberries.

Day 6:

- **Breakfast:** Smoothie with coconut milk, spinach, pineapple, and chia seeds.
- **Lunch:** Lentil and Vegetable Soup with a side of gluten-free crackers.
- **Dinner:** Grilled Shrimp Skewers with a quinoa salad and roasted Brussels sprouts.
- **Snack:** Mixed fruit bowl.

Day 7:

- **Breakfast:** Dairy-Free Yogurt Parfait with granola, raspberries, and flaxseeds.
- **Lunch:** Stuffed Sweet Potatoes with black beans, corn, avocado, and a side of sauerkraut.
- **Dinner:** Baked Tofu with stir-fried vegetables and brown rice.
- **Snack:** Apple slices with almond butter.

Sample Weekly Plan: Week 4 - Seasonal Focus

Day 1:

- **Breakfast:** Smoothie with almond milk, spinach, banana, strawberries, and chia seeds.

- **Lunch:** Seasonal Vegetable Salad with mixed greens, roasted root vegetables, quinoa, and a lemon-tahini dressing.

- **Dinner:** Grilled Chicken with a side of roasted asparagus and sweet potatoes.

- **Snack:** Fresh fruit bowl with seasonal fruits like berries and melon.

Day 2:

- **Breakfast:** Overnight Oats with almond milk, chia seeds, and seasonal fruit like pears or apples.

- **Lunch:** Hearty Vegetable Soup with carrots, celery, onions, and potatoes.

- **Dinner:** Baked Salmon with a side of quinoa and roasted Brussels sprouts.

- **Snack:** Carrot sticks with hummus.

Day 3:

- **Breakfast:** Chia Pudding with coconut milk, chia seeds, and fresh seasonal berries.

- **Lunch:** Stuffed Bell Peppers with quinoa, black beans, corn, and avocado.

- **Dinner:** Vegetable Stir-Fry with tofu, bell peppers, broccoli, and brown rice.

- **Snack:** Mixed nuts and seeds.

Day 4:

- **Breakfast:** Smoothie Bowl with almond milk, kale, banana, raspberries, and granola.

- **Lunch:** Chickpea Salad with avocado, cucumber, tomatoes, and a lemon-tahini dressing.

- **Dinner:** Baked Cod with roasted sweet potatoes and green beans.

- **Snack:** Fresh seasonal fruit with almond milk.

Day 5:

- **Breakfast:** Avocado Toast on gluten-free bread with a side of seasonal mixed fruit.

- **Lunch:** Quinoa and Black Bean Tacos with avocado, lettuce, salsa, and a side of kimchi.

- **Dinner:** Grilled Tempeh with stir-fried seasonal vegetables and rice noodles.

- **Snack:** Dairy-free yogurt with fresh seasonal fruit.

Day 6:

- **Breakfast:** Smoothie with coconut milk, spinach, pineapple, and chia seeds.

- **Lunch:** Lentil and Seasonal Vegetable Soup with a side of gluten-free crackers.

- **Dinner:** Grilled Shrimp Skewers with quinoa salad and roasted Brussels sprouts.

- **Snack:** Mixed seasonal fruit bowl.

Day 7:

- **Breakfast:** Dairy-Free Yogurt Parfait with granola, fresh seasonal fruit, and flaxseeds.

- **Lunch:** Stuffed Sweet Potatoes with black beans, corn, avocado, and a side of sauerkraut.

- **Dinner:** Baked Tofu with stir-fried seasonal vegetables and brown rice.

- **Snack:** Apple slices with almond butter.

Hydration and Gut-Friendly Beverages

Importance of Hydration

Staying hydrated is essential for overall health and plays a crucial role in maintaining a healthy digestive system. Water helps in the digestion and absorption of nutrients, supports the removal of waste, and maintains the mucosal lining of the intestines, which is essential for protecting against harmful bacteria and maintaining a balanced gut microbiome.

Benefits of Proper Hydration for Gut Health

1. **Aids Digestion:**

   o   Water helps break down food so that your body can absorb the nutrients. Proper hydration also aids in the movement of food through the intestines, preventing constipation.

2. **Supports Mucosal Lining:**

   o   Adequate water intake maintains the mucosal lining of the intestines, which protects against harmful bacteria and supports the absorption of nutrients.

3. **Promotes Regularity:**

   o   Staying hydrated helps keep stools soft and easy to pass, preventing constipation and promoting regular bowel movements.

4. **Balances Gut Microbiome:**

   o   Hydration helps maintain a healthy environment for beneficial bacteria in the gut, supporting a balanced microbiome.

5. **Detoxification:**

   o   Water assists in flushing out toxins from the body through urine and sweat, reducing the burden on the digestive system.

Recommended Daily Water Intake

While individual water needs can vary based on factors like age, sex, weight, and activity level, a general guideline is to drink at least 8-10 cups (2-2.5 liters) of water per day. It's important to listen to your body and drink more if you are active, in a hot climate, or feeling thirsty.

Gut-Friendly Beverages

In addition to water, several beverages can support gut health. These drinks provide hydration while offering additional benefits such as probiotics, anti-inflammatory properties, and essential nutrients.

Probiotic-Rich Beverages

1. **Kefir:**

   o A fermented milk drink rich in probiotics that can help balance the gut microbiome and improve digestion.

2. **Kombucha:**

   o A fermented tea containing probiotics and antioxidants that support gut health and overall wellness.

3. **Probiotic Smoothies:**

   o Smoothies made with probiotic-rich yogurt or kefir, blended with fruits and vegetables for added fiber and nutrients.

Anti-Inflammatory Beverages

1. **Turmeric Tea:**

   o Made with turmeric, ginger, and honey, this tea has anti-inflammatory properties that can soothe the digestive tract.

2. **Ginger Tea:**

   o Ginger tea aids in digestion, reduces nausea, and has anti-inflammatory effects that benefit gut health.

3. **Green Tea:**

   o Rich in antioxidants and anti-inflammatory properties, green tea can promote a healthy gut and overall health.

Hydrating Herbal Teas

1. **Peppermint Tea:**

   o Peppermint tea can help relieve digestive symptoms like bloating, gas, and indigestion.

2. **Chamomile Tea:**

   o Chamomile tea is known for its calming effects and can help soothe the digestive system and reduce inflammation.

3. **Fennel Tea:**

- Fennel tea can help alleviate digestive issues such as bloating and gas, and supports overall digestive health.

Nutritious Juices and Smoothies

1. **Green Juice:**
   - Made with leafy greens, cucumber, celery, and a touch of fruit, green juice is packed with nutrients that support gut health and hydration.

2. **Fiber-Rich Smoothies:**
   - Smoothies made with fruits, vegetables, and added fiber sources like chia seeds or flaxseeds can promote healthy digestion and regularity.

3. **Aloe Vera Juice:**
   - Aloe vera juice has soothing properties that can support digestive health and hydration.

Sample Hydration Plan

Morning:

- Start your day with a glass of warm water with lemon to kickstart digestion and hydration.
- Have a cup of green tea or a probiotic smoothie for breakfast.

Mid-Morning:

- Drink a glass of water or herbal tea like ginger or peppermint tea.

Afternoon:

- Enjoy a hydrating green juice or a glass of water with a splash of aloe vera juice.
- Have a cup of turmeric tea with lunch for its anti-inflammatory benefits.

Evening:

- Drink a glass of water or a cup of chamomile tea to relax and support digestion before bed.

Chapter 13: Lifestyle and Gut Health

Exercise and Digestion

Regular physical activity plays a significant role in maintaining digestive health and overall well-being. Exercise can help improve digestion, alleviate digestive discomfort, and support a healthy gut microbiome. Here's how exercise influences digestion and tips on incorporating it into your routine for optimal gut health:

How Exercise Affects Digestion

1. **Promotes Regular Bowel Movements:**

   o Physical activity helps stimulate the muscles of the intestines, promoting regular bowel movements and preventing constipation.

2. **Reduces Bloating and Gas:**

   o Exercise can help reduce bloating and gas by moving gas through the digestive tract more efficiently.

3. **Improves Gut Motility:**

   o Exercise enhances gut motility, the movement of food and waste through the digestive system, which aids in digestion and absorption of nutrients.

4. **Enhances Blood Flow to the Digestive Organs:**

   o Increased blood flow to the digestive organs during exercise improves their function, including digestion and nutrient absorption.

5. **Supports a Healthy Gut Microbiome:**

   o Regular exercise has been shown to positively influence the composition and diversity of gut microbiota, promoting a healthier balance of bacteria in the gut.

Types of Exercises Beneficial for Digestion

1. **Aerobic Exercise:**

   o Activities like walking, jogging, cycling, and swimming increase heart rate and breathing, promoting movement in the intestines and improving digestion.

2. **Yoga:**

- Yoga poses that involve twisting, bending, and stretching can massage the internal organs, stimulate digestion, and relieve constipation.

3. **Strength Training:**

   - Resistance exercises such as weightlifting or using resistance bands can improve overall muscle tone, including the muscles of the abdomen and core, which supports digestive function.

4. **Pilates:**

   - Pilates exercises focus on core strength, stability, and posture, which can improve digestion by supporting proper alignment of the digestive organs.

5. **Mindful Movement Practices:**

   - Practices like tai chi or qigong incorporate gentle, flowing movements that can reduce stress and promote relaxation, benefiting overall digestion.

Tips for Incorporating Exercise into Your Routine

1. **Start Slowly and Gradually Increase Intensity:**

   - Begin with activities that you enjoy and can comfortably do. Gradually increase duration and intensity as your fitness level improves.

2. **Mix Different Types of Exercises:**

   - Incorporate a variety of aerobic, strength training, and flexibility exercises to support overall health and digestion.

3. **Stay Hydrated:**

   - Drink water before, during, and after exercise to stay hydrated and support digestive processes.

4. **Mindful Eating After Exercise:**

   - Avoid heavy meals immediately before exercising. After exercise, choose nutrient-dense foods that support recovery and digestion.

5. **Listen to Your Body:**

   - Pay attention to how your body responds to exercise. If you experience discomfort or pain, modify your routine or consult with a healthcare professional.

Timing of Exercise and Digestive Health

- **Before Meals:** Light exercise before meals, such as a short walk, can stimulate appetite and prepare your digestive system for food.

- **After Meals:** Gentle activities like walking or yoga after meals can aid digestion by promoting movement in the digestive tract.

- **Consistency:** Aim for regular exercise most days of the week to experience the ongoing benefits for digestion and overall health.

Stress Management for Optimal Digestive Health

Stress can significantly impact digestive health by affecting the gut-brain axis, increasing inflammation, and altering gut motility. Managing stress effectively is crucial for maintaining a healthy digestive system and overall well-being. Here's how stress impacts digestion and effective strategies for stress management:

How Stress Affects Digestion

1. **Impact on Gut Function:**

   o Stress activates the body's "fight or flight" response, leading to decreased blood flow and oxygen to the digestive system, which can slow digestion and impair nutrient absorption.

2. **Changes in Gut Microbiota:**

   o Chronic stress can alter the composition of gut microbiota, reducing beneficial bacteria and increasing harmful bacteria, which may contribute to digestive disorders.

3. **Increased Sensitivity:**

   o Stress can heighten sensitivity in the gut, exacerbating symptoms of irritable bowel syndrome (IBS), such as abdominal pain, bloating, and diarrhea.

4. **Inflammation:**

   o Stress triggers the release of inflammatory mediators in the body, which can contribute to inflammation in the gastrointestinal tract and worsen conditions like gastritis or inflammatory bowel disease (IBD).

5. **Disrupted Gut Motility:**

   o Stress can lead to changes in gut motility, causing either constipation or diarrhea, depending on individual responses.

Effective Strategies for Stress Management

1. **Mindfulness Meditation:**

   o Practice mindfulness meditation to reduce stress levels, promote relaxation, and improve resilience to stressors. Focus on deep breathing and staying present in the moment.

2. **Yoga and Tai Chi:**

154

- o Engage in gentle exercises like yoga or tai chi, which combine physical movement with mindfulness to reduce stress and promote relaxation.

3. **Regular Physical Activity:**

   - o Participate in regular exercise, such as walking, jogging, or cycling, to release endorphins, reduce stress hormones, and improve overall mood.

4. **Deep Breathing Exercises:**

   - o Practice deep breathing exercises or diaphragmatic breathing techniques to activate the body's relaxation response and calm the mind.

5. **Progressive Muscle Relaxation (PMR):**

   - o Perform PMR exercises to systematically tense and relax muscle groups, promoting physical relaxation and reducing stress levels.

6. **Healthy Sleep Habits:**

   - o Maintain a regular sleep schedule, aim for 7-9 hours of quality sleep per night, and create a relaxing bedtime routine to support stress reduction and overall well-being.

7. **Social Support:**

   - o Connect with supportive friends, family members, or a therapist to share feelings, gain perspective, and receive emotional support during stressful times.

8. **Mindful Eating:**

   - o Practice mindful eating by focusing on enjoying and savoring each bite of food. Avoid eating in stressful situations or when distracted.

9. **Time Management and Prioritization:**

   - o Organize tasks, set realistic goals, and prioritize activities to reduce feelings of overwhelm and manage stress effectively.

10. **Limit Stressors:**

   - o Identify and limit exposure to stressful triggers when possible. Delegate tasks, set boundaries, and practice assertiveness to reduce unnecessary stress.

Incorporating Stress Management into Daily Life

- **Morning Routine:** Start your day with a few minutes of deep breathing or meditation to set a positive tone for the day.

- **Midday Breaks:** Take short breaks throughout the day to practice mindfulness, stretch, or go for a walk to recharge and manage stress levels.

- **Evening Rituals:** Wind down in the evening with a relaxing activity such as reading, listening to calming music, or taking a warm bath to promote relaxation and prepare for restful sleep.

Sleep and Gut Health

Quality sleep is crucial for overall health, including digestive wellness. Sleep influences various aspects of gut health, such as gut microbiota balance, digestion, and immune function. Here's how sleep impacts the gut and tips for improving sleep for optimal digestive health:

How Sleep Affects Digestive Health

1. **Gut Microbiota Balance:**

   o Adequate sleep supports a healthy balance of gut microbiota, promoting diversity and abundance of beneficial bacteria essential for digestion and immune function.

2. **Digestive Processes:**

   o During sleep, the body undergoes repair and restoration processes, including digestion and absorption of nutrients. Disrupted sleep can impair these functions.

3. **Gut-Brain Axis:**

   o Sleep influences the gut-brain axis, affecting gut motility, sensitivity, and the release of neurotransmitters that regulate digestion and appetite.

4. **Inflammation and Immune Response:**

   o Poor sleep patterns can lead to increased inflammation in the gastrointestinal tract and compromise immune responses, impacting gut health.

5. **Hormonal Regulation:**

   o Sleep helps regulate hormones involved in appetite control and metabolism, such as leptin and ghrelin, which can influence food intake and digestive health.

Tips for Improving Sleep for Digestive Health

1. **Establish a Consistent Sleep Schedule:**

   o Maintain a regular sleep-wake cycle by going to bed and waking up at the same time each day, even on weekends, to regulate your body's internal clock.

2. **Create a Relaxing Bedtime Routine:**

   o Develop calming bedtime rituals, such as taking a warm bath, practicing relaxation techniques like deep breathing or meditation, or reading a book to unwind before sleep.

3. **Optimize Sleep Environment:**

   o Create a sleep-conducive environment by keeping your bedroom cool, dark, and quiet. Use comfortable bedding and consider using blackout curtains or a white noise machine if needed.

4. **Limit Screen Time Before Bed:**

   o Reduce exposure to electronic devices, such as smartphones, tablets, and computers, at least an hour before bedtime to promote relaxation and melatonin production.

5. **Mindful Eating Before Bed:**

   o Avoid heavy meals, spicy foods, caffeine, and alcohol close to bedtime, as they can disrupt sleep and digestion. Opt for light, easily digestible snacks if needed.

6. **Regular Exercise:**

   o Engage in regular physical activity during the day, but avoid vigorous exercise close to bedtime, as it can be stimulating and interfere with sleep.

7. **Manage Stress:**

   o Practice stress management techniques, such as meditation, yoga, or deep breathing exercises, to alleviate tension and promote relaxation before sleep.

8. **Limit Naps:**

   o If you nap during the day, keep it short (20-30 minutes) and avoid napping late in the afternoon or evening, as it can interfere with nighttime sleep.

Incorporating Good Sleep Habits into Your Routine

- **Morning Routine:** Start your day with exposure to natural light, which helps regulate your body's sleep-wake cycle and promotes alertness during the day.

- **Daytime Breaks:** Take short breaks during the day to stretch, move around, and get some fresh air, which can help maintain energy levels and improve sleep quality at night.

- **Evening Wind-Down:** Create a calming bedtime routine that signals to your body that it's time to relax and prepare for sleep. Avoid stimulating activities and electronics.

Conversion Table

Volume

US Standard	Metric Equivalent
1 teaspoon (tsp)	5 milliliters (ml)
1 tablespoon (tbsp)	15 milliliters (ml)
1 fluid ounce (fl oz)	30 milliliters (ml)
1 cup (c)	240 milliliters (ml)
1 pint (pt)	480 milliliters (ml)
1 quart (qt)	960 milliliters (ml)
1 gallon (gal)	3.8 liters (L)

Weight

US Standard	Metric Equivalent
1 ounce (oz)	28 grams (g)
1 pound (lb)	454 grams (g)
1 pound (lb)	0.45 kilograms (kg)

Length

US Standard	Metric Equivalent
1 inch (in)	2.54 centimeters (cm)
1 foot (ft)	30.48 centimeters (cm)
1 yard (yd)	0.91 meters (m)

Temperature

US Standard	Metric Equivalent
Fahrenheit (°F)	Celsius (°C)
(°F - 32) × 5/9 = °C	(°C × 9/5) + 32 = °F

Oven Temperatures

US Standard	Metric Equivalent
250°F	120°C
300°F	150°C
350°F	180°C
400°F	200°C
450°F	230°C
500°F	260°C

Common Ingredients

Ingredient	US Standard	Metric Equivalent
All-purpose flour	1 cup	120 grams
Granulated sugar	1 cup	200 grams
Brown sugar	1 cup	220 grams
Butter	1 cup	227 grams
Milk	1 cup	240 milliliters
Water	1 cup	240 milliliters
Honey	1 cup	340 grams

This conversion table will help you seamlessly convert measurements between US standard and metric systems, ensuring your recipes are accurate and consistent, no matter where you are in the world.